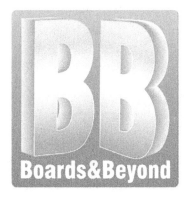

Boards and Beyond:
Hematology Slides

Slides from the Boards and Beyond Website

Jason Ryan, MD, MPH

2019 Edition

Table of Contents

Coagulation

Jason Ryan, MD, MPH

Thrombus Formation

ENDOTHELIAL DAMAGE

FIBRIN   ACTIVATED PLATELETS

THROMBUS

Vasoconstriction

- 1st line of defense against bleeding
- Occurs in response to endothelial damage
- Key mediator: endothelins
  - Proteins
  - Potent vasoconstrictors
  - Released by endothelial cells near site of damage
  - Endothelin receptor blockers used in pulmonary hypertension

---

Coagulation Factors

- Proteins synthesized in liver
- Soluble in plasma
- Activate when triggered by endothelial damage
- Form an insoluble protein: Fibrin
- Fibrin mesh prevents blood loss

Coagulation Factors

- Most circulate as inactive enzymes (zymogens)
- Many activate to become serine proteases
  - Serine: amino acid
  - Protease: cleaves proteins
  - Serine protease: protein cleavage enzyme, contains serine

Serine

Coagulation Cascade

- Sequential activation of clotting factor zymogens
- Constant low level of activation in serum
- Amplification occurs with endothelial damage
- Leads to fibrin generation

Coagulation Cascade

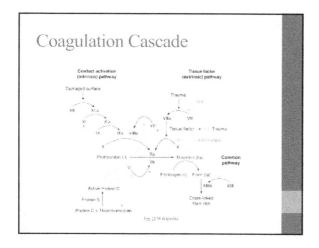

Img 2 Wikipedia

Coagulation Cascade

- Center of cascade is activation of X □ Xa
- Xa converts prothrombin (II) □ thrombin (IIa)
- Thrombin (IIa): Fibrinogen (I) □ fibrin (Ia)
- Fibrin forms plug to stop bleeding
- Activation X □ Xa makes fibrin

$$X \longrightarrow Xa$$

Coagulation Cascade

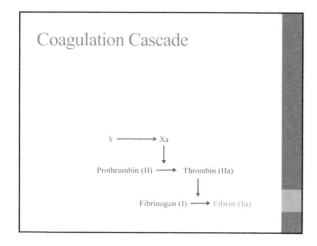

Coagulation Cascade

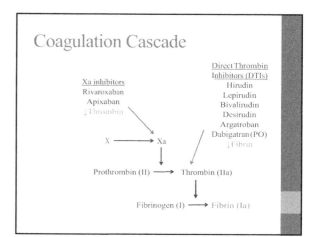

Tissue Factor

Thromboplastin

- Glycoprotein
- Constitutively expressed in sub-endothelial cells
- Not expressed by endothelial cells
- No significant contact of with circulating blood
- Exposed by endothelial damage
- Major activator of coagulation system
- Basis for Prothrombin Time and INR
  - Tissue factor added to blood sample
  - Time to form clot = PT

Coagulation Cascade

- Primary event: Exposure of tissue factor
- Interacts with factor VII □ VIIa
- TF:VIIa activates Xa

TF:VIIa

Coagulation Cascade

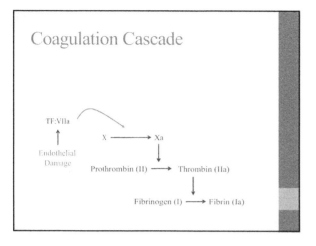

TF:VIIa

Endothelial Damage

X → Xa

Prothrombin (II) → Thrombin (IIa)

Fibrinogen (I) → Fibrin (Ia)

Thrombin

- Thrombin (IIa) makes more thrombin
- Can activate cascade (positive feedback)
  - Factor V → Va
  - Factor XI → XIa
  - Factor VIII → VIIIa
- Factor XIa activates IX → IXa
  - IX uses VIIIa as a co-factor
- IXa can also activate Xa
  - More amplification

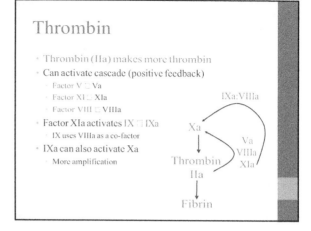

IXa:VIIIa

Xa

Va
VIIIa
XIa

Thrombin
IIa

Fibrin

Coagulation Cascade

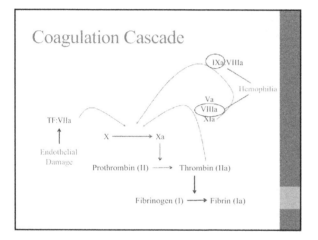

IXa:VIIIa

Va
VIIIa
XIa

Hemophilia

TF:VIIa

Endothelial Damage

X → Xa

Prothrombin (II) → Thrombin (IIa)

Fibrinogen (I) → Fibrin (Ia)

Factor VIII

- Produced in endothelial cells (not the liver)
- Circulates bound to von Willebrand Factor
  - vWF critical for platelet aggregation
  - vWF produced by endothelial cells and megakaryocytes
  - Binding to vWF increases VIII plasma halflife
- Released from vWF in response to vascular injury
  - Vascular injury → ↑ thrombin → becomes VIIIa

VIII—vWF

Multicomponent Complexes

- Two complexes for conversion X → Xa
- Three components bound together:
  - Active clotting factor functioning as enzyme
  - Co-factor
  - Substrate
- Require phospholipids and calcium
  - Phospholipid: Occur on surfaces of cells
  - TF-bearing cells or platelets
  - Calcium: Co-factor

Multicomponent Complexes

- Extrinsic Xase
  - Phospholipid: TF-bearing cells
  - Enzyme: Factor VIIa
  - Co-factor: Tissue factor
  - Substrate: Factor X

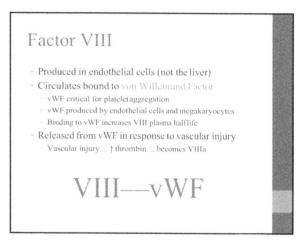

X

Ca+

TF VIIa X

Phospholipid

Xa

Multicomponent Complexes

- Intrinsic Xase
  - Phospholipid: Platelets
  - Enzyme: Factor IXa
  - Co-factor: Factor VIII (VIIIa)
  - Substrate: Factor X

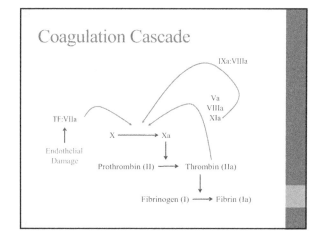

Coagulation Cascade

Coagulation Cascade

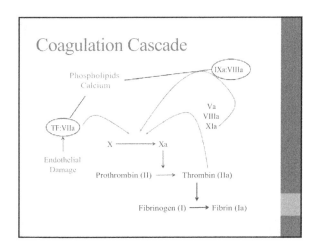

Calcium

- Factor IV
- Required for clot formation
- Activated platelets release calcium
- EDTA binds calcium in blood samples
- Prevents clotting

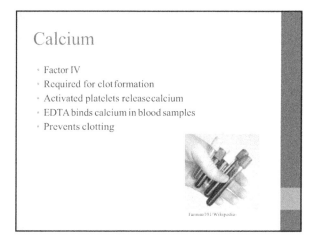

Fammm101/Wikipedia·

Factor XIII

- Crosslinks fibrin
- Stabilizes fibrin plug
- Absence of XIII ☐ inadequate clot formation
- Requires calcium as co-factor
- Activated by thrombin (IIa) formation

Coagulation Cascade

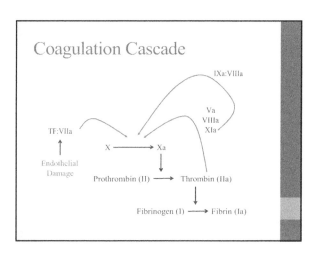

Coagulation Cascade

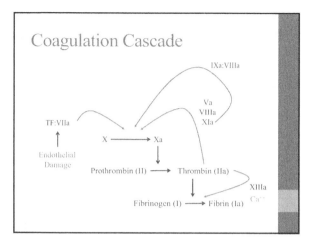

Factor XII
Hageman factor

- Can activate factor XI (XIa)
- Physiologic significance unclear
- Important for testing of coagulation system
- Activated by contact with negatively charges
- Factor XII □ XIIa via contact with silica
- Basis for partial thromboplastin time (PTT)

$$XII \longrightarrow XIIa$$
$$XI \longrightarrow XIa$$

Coagulation Cascade

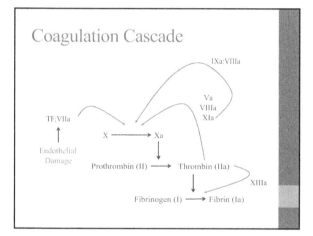

Coagulation Cascade

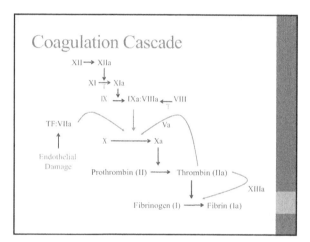

Coagulation Cascade

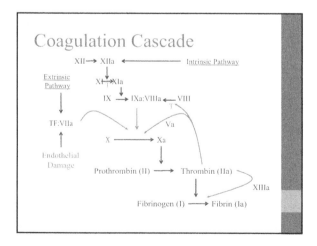

Coagulation Cascade

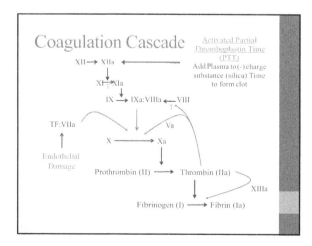

Activated Partial Thromboplastin Time (PTT)
Add Plasma to (-) charge substance (silica) Time to form clot

5

Coagulation Cascade

Prothrombin Time (PT)
Add Plasma to TF
Time to form clot

```
            ↓
         TF:VIIa                              Va
                    X ────→ Xa
       Endothelial
        Damage
              Prothrombin (II) ────→ Thrombin (IIa)
                                        ↓              XIIIa
                      Fibrinogen (I) ────→ Fibrin (Ia)
```

Intrinsic Pathway
Contact Pathway

- Requires kinins for normal function
- Kinins = peptide hormones/signaling molecules
- Short half lives
- Circulate as inactive precursors: kininogens
- Activated by kallikreins
- Kinins link coagulation with inflammation

Intrinsic Pathway
Kinin System

- Bradykinin
  - Vasodilator
  - Increases vascular permeability
  - Pain
- Degraded by angiotensin converting enzyme (ACE)
  - ACE inhibitors can raise bradykinin levels
  - Dangerous side effect: angioedema
- Also degraded by C1 inhibitor (complement system)
  - C1 inhibitor deficiency ☐ hereditary angioedema

Intrinsic Pathway
Factor XII

- Activates clotting and produces bradykinin
- Requires PK, HMWK for normal function

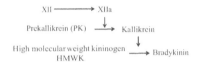

```
   XII ──────→ XIIa
                  ↓
Prekallikrein (PK) ──→ Kallikrein
                              ↓
High molecular weight kininogen ──→ Bradykinin
        HMWK
```

Prekallikrein Deficiency

- Rare condition
- Results in markedly prolonged PTT
- XII cannot activate normally
- No bleeding problems

```
   XII ──────→ XIIa
                  ↓
Prekallikrein (PK) ──→ Kallikrein
                              ↓
High molecular weight kininogen ──→ Bradykinin
        HMWK
```

Kinin System
Key Points

- Activated by factor XII
- Link between coagulation and inflammation
- Bradykinin
  - ACE inhibitors
  - Hereditary angioedema
- Prekallikrein Deoiciency: ↑PTT

Coagulation Inhibitors

- Important deactivators of coagulation
  - Antithrombin III
  - Proteins C and S
  - Tissue factor pathway inhibitor

Antithrombin III

- Serpin (inhibitor of serine proteases)
- Inhibits serine proteases: factors II, VII, IX, X, XI, XII
- Produced by liver
- Activated by endothelium
  - Endothelium makes heparan sulfate molecules
  - Activate antithrombin
  - Basis for role of heparin drug therapy
- Deficiency: Hypercoagulable state

Proteins C and S

- Glycoproteins synthesized in liver
- Protein C: zymogen
- Active form: activated protein C (APC)
- APC primarily inactivates factors Va and VIIIa

Proteins C and S

- Protein C activated by thrombomodulin
  - Cell membrane protein
  - Found on endothelial cells
- Thrombomodulin binds thrombin
  - Complex activates protein C to APC

Proteins C and S

- APC requires protein S as co-factor
- Protein S circulates in active form (not a zymogen)

Thrombomodulin: Thrombin

Protein C ⟶ APC

Inactivation
Va, VIIIa

Protein S

TFPI

Tissue factor pathway inhibitor

- Inactivates Xa via two mechanisms
  - Directly binds Xa
  - Binds TF/FVIIa complex ⟶ prevents X activation
- Plasma levels increased with heparin administration
  - May contribute to antithrombotic effect

Plasminogen and Plasmin

- Plasminogen synthesized by liver (zymogen)
- Converted to active enzyme: plasmin
- Main role of plasmin is breakdown of fibrin
  - Broad substrate specificity
  - Also degrades clotting factors, fibrinogen

Plasminogen Activators

- Tissue plasminogen activator (tPA) and urokinase
  - Synthesized by endothelial and other cells
  - Used as drug therapy for acute MI and stroke
  - Streptokinase: Streptococcal protein; activates plasminogen

FDPs and D-dimer

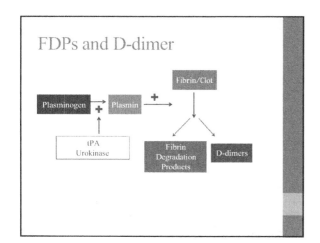

FDPs and D-dimer

- Fibrinogen has two domains: E (central) and D (side)
- Crosslinking of fibrin (XIII) creates E linked two Ds

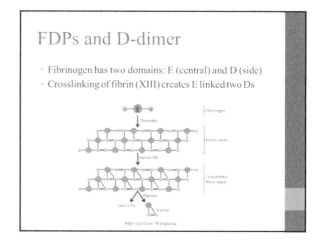

FDPs and D-dimer

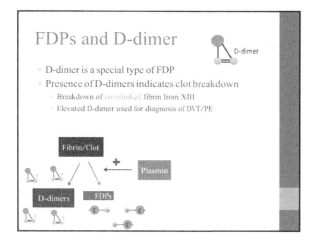

- D-dimer is a special type of FDP
- Presence of D-dimers indicates clot breakdown
  - Breakdown of crosslinked fibrin from XIII
  - Elevated D-dimer used for diagnosis of DVT/PE

FDPs and D-dimer

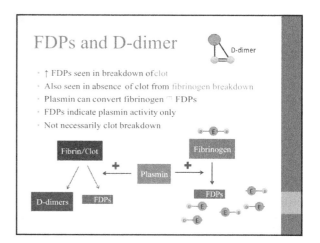

- ↑ FDPs seen in breakdown of clot
- Also seen in absence of clot from fibrinogen breakdown
- Plasmin can convert fibrinogen → FDPs
- FDPs indicate plasmin activity only
- Not necessarily clot breakdown

Primary Fibrinolysis

- Rarely phenomena: Plasmin overactive
- Causes ↑ FDP with normal D-dimer
  - "Hyperfibrinolysis"
  - Plasmin breakdown of fibrinogen (not fibrin) ⊐ FDPs
  - No clot or crosslinked fibrin ⊐ No d-dimers
  - Plasmin can deplete clotting factors
  - Increased PT/PTT with bleeding (like DIC)
  - Prostate cancer: release of urokinase
  - Cirrhosis: Loss of alpha2 antiplasmin from liver

FDPs and D-dimer
Key Points

- Clot breakdown: FDPs and D-dimers
- Hyperfibrinolysis: FDPs with normal D-dimer levels
- ↑ D-dimer used to diagnose thrombotic disorders
- Elevated levels seen in DVT/PE
  - Sensitive but not specific
  - Elevated in many other disorders

Vitamin K

- Required for synthesis of many clotting factors
  - "Vitamin K dependent clotting factors"
- Vitamin K dependent factors: II, VII, IX, X, C, S
- Vitamin K deficiency: bleeding
- Warfarin: Vitamin K antagonist

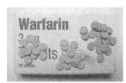

Gonegonegone /Wikipedia

ESR
Erythrocyte Sedimentation Rate

- Rate of RBC sedimentation in test tube
  - Normal 0-22 mm/hr for men; 0-29 mm/hr for women
- Increased in inflammatory conditions

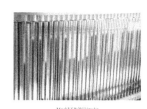

MechESR/Wikipedia

ESR
Erythrocyte Sedimentation Rate

- ESR increased by "acute phase reactants" in plasma
  - Serum proteins that rise in inflammation or tissue injury
  - Driven by cytokines
  - Most come from liver
- Key acute phase reactants
  - Fibrinogen
  - Ferritin
  - C-reactive protein (binds bacteria; activates complement)

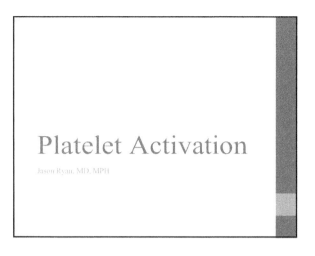

Platelet Activation

Jason Ryan, MD, MPH

Thrombus Formation

ENDOTHELIAL DAMAGE

FIBRIN   ACTIVATED PLATELETS

THROMBUS

Platelets

- Small cells derived from megakaryocytes
- Do not contain a nucleus
- Short lifespan: about 8-10 days
- Production regulated by thrombopoietin (TPO)
  - Glycoprotein produced mostly in liver

Graham Beards/Wikipedia

Platelets

- Aid in hemostasis after vascular injury
- Circulate in "inactive" form
- Can "activate" due to:
  - Endothelial injury
  - Stimuli from other activated platelets
- Activated platelets seal damaged vessels

Platelets Actions

- Adhesion to sub-endothelium
- Aggregation: Platelet-platelet binding
- Secretion: Release of granule contents
- Net result: Seal openings in vascular tree

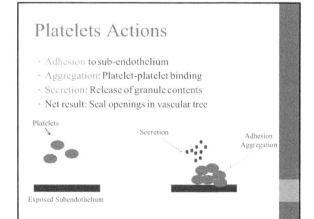

Von Willebrand Factor

- Large glycoprotein
- Synthesized by endothelial cells and megakaryocytes
  - Stored in Weibel-Palade bodies in endothelial cells
- Present in platelets (stored in alpha granules)
- Some found in plasma
- Released on vascular injury
  - Activated platelets degranulate
  - Endothelial cells release vWF

Von Willebrand Factor

- Several roles in hemostasis
- #1: Carrier protein for factor VIII
  - Factor VIII released in presence of thrombin (VIIIa)
- #2: Binds platelets to damaged endothelium
- #3: Binds activated platelets together (aggregation)

VIII—vWF

Membrane Glycoproteins

- Glycoproteins (amino acids and glucose molecules)
- Found on surface of platelets
- Interact with other structures/molecules
- Important for hemostasis
- GPIb, GPIIb/IIIa

Platelets Actions

- Adhesion to sub-endothelium
- Aggregation: Platelet-platelet binding
- Secretion: Release of granule contents

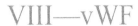

Platelet Adhesion

- Vascular damage: exposure of collagen
- Subendothelial collagen binds vWF
- vWF binds GPIb on platelets

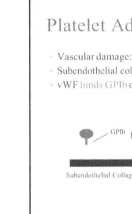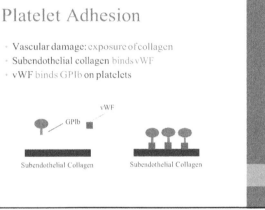

Platelet Aggregation

- Mediated by GPIIb/IIIa receptor
  - Most abundant surface receptor on platelets
- Platelet activation ☐ GPIIb/IIIa changes conformation
  - Becomes capable of binding
  - Will not bind when platelets are inactive
  - "Inside-out" signaling (cell activity ☐ altered receptor)

Platelet Aggregation

- GPIIb/IIIa binds fibrinogen or vWF
- Links platelets together (aggregation)
- Basis for IIB/IIIA receptor blocking drugs

Platelet Secretion

- Platelets activated by:
  - Binding to subendothelial collagen
  - Stimulation by activating substances
- Secretion of stored activators ▢ more activation

Secretion

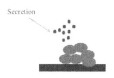

Platelet Granules

- Two types of platelet granules: alpha and dense
- Contents promote hemostasis
- Released on activation by:
  - Platelet binding to collagen
  - Granule contents from other platelets

Dr Graham Beards/Wikipedia

Platelet Granules

- Alpha granules (most abundant)
  - Fibrinogen
  - von Willebrand factor
  - platelet factor 4
- Dense granules
  - ADP
  - Calcium
  - Serotonin

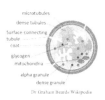

Dr Graham Beards/Wikipedia

Platelet Factor 4
PF4

- Released from alpha granules
- Binds to endothelial cells
- Numerous biologic effects described
- Heparin induced thrombocytopenia
  - Rare, life-threatening effect of heparin administration
  - Antibodies formed to PF4 complexed with heparin
  - Antibodies bind PF4-heparin ▢ platelet activation
  - Diffuse thrombosis
  - Low platelets from consumption

Serotonin

- Stored in dense granules
- Released on platelet activation
- Basis for serotonin release assay
  - Diagnostic test for HIT
  - Donor platelets radiolabeled with ^{14}C-serotonin
  - Patient serum and heparin added
  - HIT antibodies ▢ excessive serotonin release

Adenosine Diphosphate
ADP

- Released from dense granules
- Also released by red blood cells when damaged
- Binds to two G-protein receptors: $P2Y_1$ and $P2Y_{12}$
- Binding leads to ↓ cAMP formation
  - ↑ cAMP blocks platelet activation
  - Phosphodiesterase inhibitors ▢ ↑ cAMP

Adenosine Diphosphate
ADP

- $P2Y_1$
  - Calcium release, change in platelet shape
- $P2Y_{12}$
  - Platelet degranulation, ↑ aggregation
- Many $P2Y_{12}$ receptor blocking drugs
  - "ADP receptor blockers"
  - Inhibit platelet activity
  - Clopidogrel, prasugrel, ticlopidine, ticagrelor

Thromboxane A2
TXA2

- Powerful platelet activator
- TXA2 receptors found on platelets
- Basis for aspirin therapy

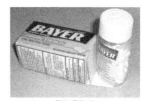

Shizhao/Wikipedia

Thromboxane A2
TXA2

- Lipids in cell membranes ▢ arachidonic acid (AA)
  - Enzyme: phospholipase A2
  - Occurs in endothelial cells near damaged endothelium
  - AA released at sites of vascular injury
  - Also stored in platelets
- AA converted by platelets to TXA2
  - Enzyme: Cyclooxygenase (COX)
- Aspirin: Inhibits COX ▢ ↓ TXA2 ▢ platelet activation

Bleeding Time

- Test of platelet function
- Small cut to patient's arm
- Filter paper applied/removed until bleeding stops
- Rarely done in modern era

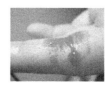

Crystal/Flikr

Hypercoagulable States

Jason Ryan, MD, MPH

Hypercoagulable States

- Predisposition to venous or arterial thrombi
- Often DVT/PEs ("Venous thromboembolism")

  - Stroke
  - Myocardial infarction
  - Ischemic limb

Virchow's Triad

- Endothelial damage
  - Endothelium makes numerous natural anticoagulants
  - Nitric oxide, prostaglandins, antithrombin, tPA, APC
- Stasis of blood
  - Normal blood flow prevents pooling of clotting factors
- Hypercoagulability
  - Conditions that increase clot formation

Hypercoagulable States

- Post-op
  - Hypercoagulable (inflammation from surgery)
  - Stasis (immobile)
  - Endothelial damage (surgery)
- Fall/Hip Fracture/Trauma
  - Hypercoagulable (inflammation from trauma)
  - Stasis (immobility)
  - Endothelial damage (trauma)
- Long plane flights
  - Stasis (immobility)

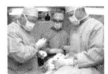

Wikipedia/Public Domain

Hypercoagulable States

- Malignancy
  - Some tumors produce pro-coagulants (i.e. tissue factor)
  - Adenocarcinomas: some data that mucin is thrombogenic
- Normal cells may produce pro-coagulants
  - Reaction to presence/growth of tumor
- Decreased activity, surgery, bed rest

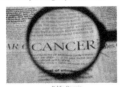

Public Domain

Hypercoagulable States

- Pregnancy
  - Probably evolved to protect against blood loss at delivery
  - Many clotting factor levels change
  - Increased fibrinogen
  - Decreased protein S
  - Fetus also obstructs venous return → DVTs common
- Oral contraceptive pills (OCPs)
  - Estrogen increases production coagulation factors

Hypercoagulable States

- Elevated homocysteine (amino acid)
- Associated with arterial and venous clots
- High levels may cause:
  - Endothelial injury
  - Activation of some clotting factors
- Elevated levels caused by:
  - Folate/B12/B6 deficiency
  - Homocystinuria (cystathionine beta synthase deficiency)
- Levels lowered by folate
  - Most clinical trials of folate did not show benefit

$$HS \diagup\diagdown\diagup \begin{smallmatrix} O \\ \| \\ \end{smallmatrix}\!\! - OH$$
$$NH_2$$

Hypercoagulable States

- Nephrotic syndrome
  - Multiple mechanisms
  - Loss of anti-clotting factors in urine (ATIII)

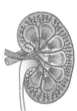

Holly Fischer/Wikipedia

Hypercoagulable States

- Smoking
  - Associated with atherosclerosis and MI/Stroke
  - Some data linking smoking to DVT/PE
  - Evidence that smoking increases fibrinogen levels

Pixabay/Public Domain

Inherited Thrombophilia

- Inherited hypercoagulable states
- Genetic tendencies to VTE
- Most involve coagulation pathway defects
- All associated with venous clots (DVT/PE)

Hypercoagulable Condition
Factor V Leiden Mutation
Prothrombin gene mutation
Antithrombin deficiency
Protein C/S deficiency

Factor V Leiden Mutation

- Named for Leiden, Netherlands
- Abnormal factor V
- Not inactivated by activated protein C (APC)
- Factor V remains active longer □ hypercoagulability

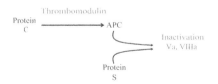

Factor V Leiden Mutation

- Point mutation in factor V gene
  - Guanine to adenine change
- Result: Single amino acid change
  - Arginine to glutamine substitution
  - Position 506 in factor V

Prothrombin Gene Mutation

- Prothrombin 20210 gene mutation
  - Guanine to adenine change in prothrombin gene
  - Occurs at nucleotide 20210
- Heterozygous carriers: 30% ↑ prothrombin levels

Prothrombin (II) ⟶ Thrombin (IIa)

↓

Fibrinogen (I) ⟶ Fibrin (Ia)

Antithrombin III Deficiency

- Inherited deficiencies due to gene mutations
- Acquired deficiencies:
  - Impaired production (liver disease)
  - Protein losses (nephrotic syndrome)
  - Consumption (DIC)
- Classically presents as heparin resistance
  - Escalating dose of heparin
  - No/little change in PTT

Protein C or S Deficiency

- Protein C: associated with warfarin skin necrosis
- Initial warfarin therapy ⬚ ↓ protein C (short half life)
- If protein C deficient ⬚ marked ↓ protein C
- Result: thrombosis of skin tissue
- Large dark, purple skin lesions

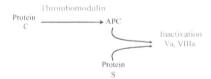

Thrombomodulin

Protein C ⟶ APC

Inactivation Va, VIIIa

Protein S

Antiphospholipid Syndrome

- Caused by antiphospholipid antibodies
- Occur in association with lupus or as primary disease

Antiphospholipid Syndrome

- Three important clinical consequences of antibodies
- "Antiphospholipid syndrome"
  - #1: Increased risk of venous and arterial thrombosis
    - Most commonly DVT
    - Also CNS: stroke
    - Recurrent fetal loss
  - #2: Increased PTT
  - #3: False positive syphilis (RPR/VDRL)

Antiphospholipid Syndrome

- Anti-cardiolipin
  - False positive RPR/VDRL
    Syphilis also produces these antibodies
- "Lupus anticoagulant"
  - Interferes with PTT test (silica activation of XII)
  - False elevation
- Anti-β2 glycoprotein

Antiphospholipid Syndrome
Antibody Detection

- Anti-cardiolipin, Anti-β2 glycoprotein
  - Enzyme-linked immunosorbent assay (ELISA) testing
- "Lupus anticoagulant"
  - Detected indirectly through coagulation assays

Lupus Anticoagulant

Coagulation cascade requires phospholipids

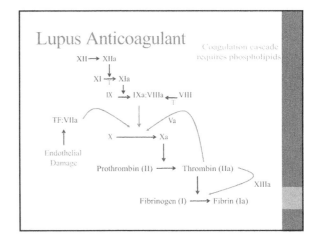

Lupus Anticoagulant
PTT Testing

- Lupus anticoagulant binds phospholipid □ ↑PTT

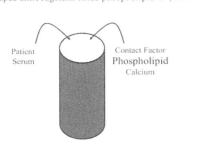

Patient Serum

Contact Factor
Phospholipid
Calcium

Lupus Anticoagulant
Mixing Study

- Can show presence of lupus anticoagulant (inhibitor)

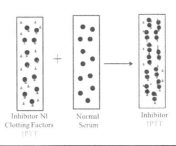

Inhibitor Nl
Clotting Factors
↑PTT

Normal
Serum

Inhibitor
↑PTT

Lupus Anticoagulant
Mixing Study

- Clotting factor deficiency: PTT corrects to normal
- Clotting factors ~50% normal □ normal PT/PTT

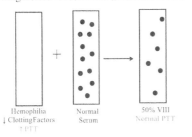

Hemophilia
↓ Clotting Factors
↑PTT

Normal
Serum

50% VIII
Normal PTT

Lupus Anticoagulant
Other Tests

- Only ~50% patients with LA have ↑PTT
- Other coagulation tests sometimes used
  - Dilute Russell viper venom time
  - Kaolin clotting time
- Time to clot will be prolonged if LA present
- Time to clot will not correct with mixing study

Antiphospholipid Antibodies
Testing

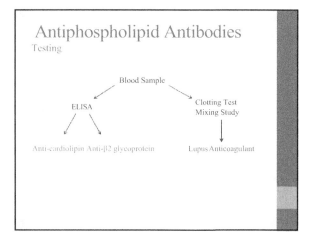

Antiphospholipid Syndrome

- Syndrome = one laboratory plus one clinical criteria
- Lab criteria (2 positive results >12 weeks apart):
  - Lupus anticoagulant
  - Anti-cardiolipin
  - Anti-β2-glycoprotein
- Clinical criteria:
  - Arterial or venous thrombosis
  - Fetal death after 10 weeks of normal fetus
  - >=3 consecutive fetal losses before 10 weeks

Hypercoagulable Workup

- Panel of tests for hypercoagulable states
- Sometimes performed in:
  - Unprovoked DVT/PE
  - Stroke/MI at an early age
- Controversial
  - Expensive
  - Rarely changes management
  - Few data on management of identified states
  - Risk of bleeding with indefinite anticoagulation
- Some tests altered by thrombus or blood thinners

Hypercoagulable Workup

- Antithrombin level
- Protein C and S levels
- Factor V Leiden gene mutation
- Prothrombin gene mutation
- Antiphospholipid antibodies
- Cancer screening

Coagulopathies

Jason Ryan, MD, MPH

Bleeding Disorders

- Abnormal coagulation cascade
  - Hemophilia, Vitamin K deficiency
- Abnormal platelets
  - Bernard-Soulier, Glanzmann's Thrombasthenia
  - ITP, TTP

- Mixed Disorders
  - Von Willebrand Disease, DIC, Liver disease

Bleeding Time

- Test of platelet function
- Small cut to patient's arm
- Filter paper applied/removed until bleeding stops
- Rarely done in modern era

PTT
Activated Partial Thromboplastin Time

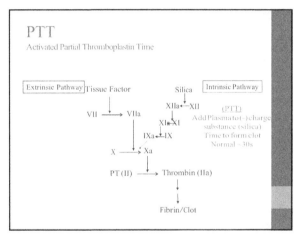

PT
Prothrombin Time

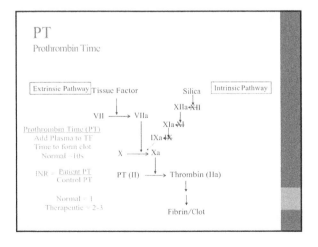

Thrombin Time

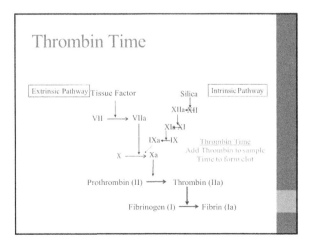

Type of Bleeding

- Abnormal platelets
  - Mucosal bleeding, skin bleeding, petechiae
- Abnormal coagulation factors
  - Joint bleeding, deep tissue bleeding

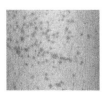

Hektor, Wikipedia

Hemophilias

- X-linked recessive diseases
- Gene mutations: Run in families; also occur de novo
- Hemophilia A: Deficiency of factor VIII
- Hemophilia B: Deficiency of factor IX
  - Also called Christmas disease

Alexei Nikolaevich

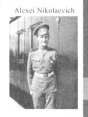

Hemophilias

- Present with spontaneous or easy bruising
- Recurrent joint bleeds is common presentation
- Screening: PTT will be prolonged
  - Factors VIII, IX both part of intrinsic pathway
- PT, bleeding time, platelet count all normal

Coagulation Cascade

$$XII \rightarrow XIIa$$

$$XI \rightarrow XIa$$

$$IX \rightarrow IXa:VIIIa \leftarrow VIII$$

TF:VIIa

Va

Endothelial Damage

$$X \rightarrow Xa$$

$$Prothrombin\ (II) \rightarrow Thrombin\ (IIa)$$

XIIIa

$$Fibrinogen\ (I) \rightarrow Fibrin\ (Ia)$$

Ca+

VIIIa IX X

Phospholipid

Hemophilias
Treatment

- Replacement factor VIII and IX

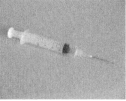

Riggwelter, commons.wiki

Hemophilias
Treatment

- Desmopressin (dDAVP)
  - Used in mild hemophilia A
  - Analogue of vasopressin (ADH) with no pressor activity
  - Increases vWF and factor VIII levels
  - Releases VIII from Weibel-Palade bodies(endothelial cells)

Desmopressin

- Also has vasodilating properties
- Key side effects: flushing, headache
- Other uses:
  - von Willebrand disease
  - Central diabetes insipidus (mimics ADH)
  - Bedwetting (decreases urine volume)

Hemophilias
Treatment

- Aminocaproic acid
  - Antifibrinolytic drug
  - Inhibits plasminogen activation ⁻ plasmin
  - Less breakdown of formed clots

Cryoprecipitate
"Cryo"

- Obsolete therapy for hemophilia A
- Precipitate that forms when FFP is thawed
- Separated from plasma by centrifugation
- Contains factor VIII, fibrinogen
- Also factor XIII and von Willebrand factor (VWF)
- Often used as source of fibrinogen
  - DIC
  - Massive trauma with blood transfusions

Coagulation Factor Inhibitors

- Antibodies
- Inhibit activity or increase clearance of clotting factor
- Inhibitors of factor VIII most common
- Often occur in association with:
  - Malignancy
  - Post-partum
  - Autoimmune disorders
- Can be treated with prednisone

Martin Brändli /Wikipedia

Coagulation Factor Inhibitors

- Can present similar to hemophilia
  - Deficient activity of VIII ⁻ bleeding
  - Prolonged PTT
- Mixing study will differentiate from hemophilia A

Mixing Study

- Clotting factors ~50% normal ⁻ normal PT/PTT

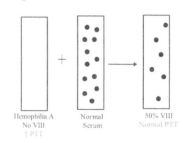

Hemophilia A	Normal	50% VIII
No VIII	Serum	Normal PTT
↑ PTT		

Mixing Study

- Clotting factors ~50% normal ⬜ normal PT/PTT

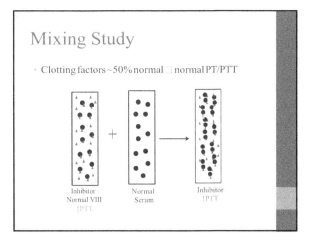

Inhibitor
Normal VIII
↑PTT

Normal
Serum

Inhibitor
↑PTT

Vitamin K Deficiency

- Results in bleeding
- Deficiency of vitamin K-dependent factors
  - II, VII, IX, X
- Key lab findings:
  - Elevated PT/INR
  - Can see elevated PTT (less sensitive)
  - Normal bleeding time

Vitamin K Deficiency

- Dietary deficiency rare
- GI bacteria produce sufficient quantities
- Common causes:
  - Warfarin
  - Antibiotics (deplete GI bacteria)
  - Newborns (sterile GI tract)
  - Malabsorption (Vitamin K is fat soluble)

Blood Transfusion

- Large volume transfusions ⬜ dilution clotting factors
- Packed RBCs: devoid of plasma/platelets
  - Removed after collection
- Saline or IVF: No clotting factors
- Treated with fresh frozen plasma

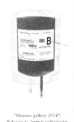

"Hansen gallery 2014".
Wikiversity Journal of Medicine.

Liver Disease

- Loss of clotting factors
  - Advanced liver disease ⬜ ↓ clotting factor synthesis
  - Most clotting factors produced in liver
  - Exception: Factor VIII produced in endothelial cells
  - PT more sensitive to liver disease (vitamin K)
- Thrombocytopenia also common
  - Decreased hepatic synthesis of thrombopoietin
  - Platelet sequestration in spleen from portal hypertension

Platelet Disorders

Jason Ryan, MD, MPH

Bleeding Disorders

- Abnormal coagulation
  - Hemophilia, Vitamin K deficiency
- Abnormal platelets
  - Bernard-Soulier
  - Glanzmann's Thrombasthenia
  - Uremia
- Mixed Disorders
  - Von Willebrand Disease, DIC

Type of Bleeding

- Abnormal platelets
  - Mucosal bleeding, skin bleeding, petechiae
- Abnormal coagulation factors
  - Joint bleeding, deep tissue bleeding

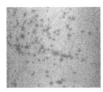

Hektor/Wikipedia

Bleeding Time

- Test of platelet function
- Small cut to patient's arm
- Filter paper applied/removed until bleeding stops
- Rarely done in modern era

Inherited Platelet Disorders

Inherited Platelet Disorders

Glanzman's Thrombasthenia Deficiency IIB/IIIA

Bernard-Soulier Deficiency IB

Wiscott-Aldrich Immunodeficiency

Glanzmann's Thrombasthenia

- Autosomal recessive disorder
- Functional deficiency of GPIIb/IIIa receptors
- Bleeding, often epistaxis
- Key diagnostic finding:
  - Prolonged bleeding time
  - Blood smear: Isolated platelets (no clumping)
  - Absent platelet aggregation in response to stimuli
  - Abnormal platelet aggregometry
  - Platelets mixed with ADP, arachidonic acid

Bernard-Soulier Syndrome

- Autosomal recessive disorder
- Deficiency of GPIb platelet receptors
- Platelets cannot bind vWF
- Also results in large platelets
- Bleeding, often epistaxis or menorrhagia
- Key lab findings:
  - Prolonged bleeding time
  - Thrombocytopenia
  - Large platelets on blood smear

Giant Platelets

- Can be seen in association with thrombocytopenia
- Caused by rare inherited disorders
  - Bernard-Soulier, others

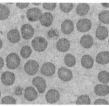

Bobjgalindo/Wikipedia

Wiskott-Aldrich Syndrome

- Immunodeficiency syndrome of infants
- X linked disorder of WAS gene (WAS protein)
  - Necessary for T-cell cytoskeleton maintenance
- Triad:
  - Immune dysfunction
  - ↓ platelets
  - Eczema

ITP
Idiopathic thrombocytopenic purpura

- Disorder of decreased platelet survival
- Commonly caused by anti-GPIIB/IIIA antibodies
- Consumption splenic macrophages

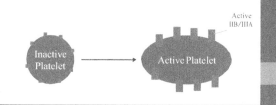

ITP
Idiopathic thrombocytopenic purpura

- Diagnosis of exclusion
  - Rule out other causes of bone marrow suppression
- Treatment:
  - Steroids
  - IVIG (blocks Fc receptors in macrophages)
  - Splenectomy

TTP
Thrombotic thrombocytopenic purpura

- Disorder of small vessel thrombus formation
- Consumes platelets ☐ thrombocytopenia
- ↓ activity of vWF cleaving protease ADAMTS13

Von Willebrand Factor
Multimers

- vWF synthesized a protein monomer
  - Occurs in endothelial cells and megakaryocytes
- Monomers link in endoplasmic reticulum ☐ dimers
- vWF dimers move to Golgi ☐ multimers

Von Willebrand Factor
Multimers

- Large multimers stored:
  - Endothelial Weibel–Palade bodies
  - Platelet α-granules
- Large multimers can obstruct blood flow
- ADAMTS13 prevents obstruction
  - Enzyme (metalloprotease)
  - Breaks down multimers of vWF
  - Prevents thrombotic occlusion

ADAMTS13

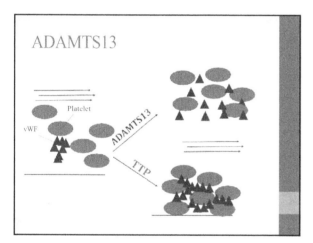

TTP
Cause

- Severe ADAMTS13 deficiency
  - Usually <10% normal activity
- Usual cause: acquired autoantibody to ADAMTS13
- Result: vWF multimers in areas of high shear stress
- Obstruction small vessels

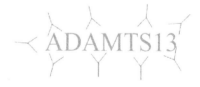

MAHA
Microangiopathic hemolytic anemia

- Hemolytic anemia (↑LDH, ↓ haptoglobin)
- Caused by shearing of RBCs as they pass through thrombi in small vessels
- Blood smear: schistocytes
- Seen in:
  - TTP
  - HUS
  - DIC

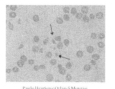

Paulo Henrique Orlandi Mourao

TTP
Thrombotic thrombocytopenic purpura

- Fever
  - Inflammation from small vessel occlusion and tissue damage
- Neurological symptoms
  - Headache, confusion, seizures
- Renal failure
- Petechiae and bleeding

TTP
Thrombotic thrombocytopenic purpura

- Lab tests:
  - Hemolytic anemia
  - Thrombocytopenia
  - Schistocytes on blood smear
- PT/PTT should be normal
  - Contrast with DIC
- May see elevated d-dimer

TTP
Treatment

- Plasma exchange: removes antibodies
- Platelet counts monitored to determine efficacy

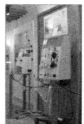

Mr Vaccha/Wikipedia

Hemolytic Uremic Syndrome
HUS

- Many similarities with TTP
- Also caused by platelet-rich thrombi in small vessels
- MAHA, thrombocytopenia, acute kidney injury
  - Usually no fever or CNS symptoms
  - Renal thrombi ☐ kidney injury
- Commonly seen in children
- Commonly follow GI infection E. Coli O157:H7
  - Shiga-like toxin causes microthrombi

DIC
Disseminated Intravascular Coagulation

- Widespread activation of clotting cascade
- Diffuse thrombi (platelets/fibrin) ☐ ischemia
- Consumption of clotting factors and platelets
- Destruction of red blood cells ☐ anemia

DIC
Disseminated Intravascular Coagulation

- Occurs secondary to another process
- Obstetrical emergencies
  - Amniotic fluid contains tissue factor
  - DIC seen in conjunction with amniotic fluid embolism
- Sepsis
  - Endotoxin --> activates coagulation cascade
  - Cytokines

DIC
Disseminated Intravascular Coagulation

- Leukemia
  - Especially acute promyelocytic leukemia (APML)
  - Cancer: well-described hypercoagulable state
  - Excess coagulation: DIC
- Rattlesnake bites
  - Thrombin-like glycoproteins within venom
  - Diffuse activation of clotting

Andy king50/Wikipedia

DIC
Disseminated Intravascular Coagulation

- Elevated PT/PTT/Thrombin time
  - Consumption of factors
- Low platelets
  - Consumption of platelets
- Low fibrinogen (consumption)
- Microangiopathic hemolytic anemia
  - Low RBC (anemia)
  - Schistocytes on blood smear
- Elevated D-dimer

DIC
Disseminated Intravascular Coagulation

- Treatment: underlying disorder
- Fresh frozen plasma: replace clotting factors
- RBCs, platelets
- Cryoprecipitate (for low fibrinogen)

ITP, TTP, HUS, DIC

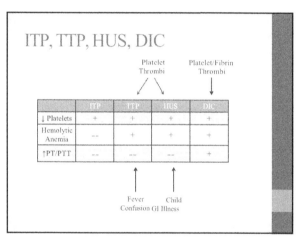

	ITP	TTP	HUS	DIC
↓ Platelets	+	+	+	+
Hemolytic Anemia	--	+	+	+
↑PT/PTT	--	--	--	+

Uremia

- Renal dysfunction ☐ bleeding
- Poor aggregation and adhesion of platelets
- Caused by uremic toxins in plasma
  - Uremic platelets work normally in normal serum
- Prolonged bleeding time
- Normal platelet count
- Normal coagulation testing

Thrombocytopenia

- Decreased production of platelets
  - Chemotherapy, leukemia
  - Sepsis (bone marrow suppression)
- Platelet sequestration
  - Splenomegaly
  - Portal hypertension
- Platelet destruction
  - ITP, TTP

Thrombocytopenia

- Normal platelet count: 150,000/ml to 400,000/ml
- Bleeding occurs when <10,000
- Treatment: Platelet transfusions

Von Willebrand Disease

- Deficient function of von Willebrand Factor
  - Large glycoprotein
  - Synthesized by endothelial cells and megakaryocytes
  - Present in platelets
- Two key roles in hemostasis
  - Carrier of factor VIII (intrinsic coagulation pathway)
  - Binds platelets to endothelium and other platelets

Von Willebrand Disease

- Most common inherited bleeding disorder
  - Affects up to 1 percent of population
- Gene mutations □ ↓ level or function of vWF
  - Most cases autosomal dominant (males=females)

Von Willebrand Disease

- Usually mild, non-life-threatening bleeding
- Easy bruising
- Skin bleeding
- Prolonged bleeding from mucosal surfaces
  - Severe nosebleeds
  - Menorrhagia

Von Willebrand Disease
Diagnosis

- Normal platelet count
- Normal PT
- Increased PTT (depending on severity)
  - Usually no joint/deep tissue bleeding
- Increased bleeding time

Von Willebrand Disease
Diagnosis

- Ristocetin cofactor activity assay
- Ristocetin: antibiotic off market due to ↓platelets
- Binds vWF and platelet glycoprotein Ib
- Causes platelet aggregation if vWF present

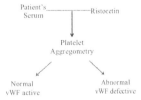

Von Willebrand Disease
Treatment

- vWF concentrate
- Desmopressin
  - Increases vWF and factor VIII levels
  - Releases vWF from endothelial cells
- Aminocaproic acid
  - Antifibrinolytic drug
  - Inhibits plasminogen activation □ plasmin
  - Less breakdown of formed clots

Heyde's Syndrome

- GI bleeding **associated with** aortic stenosis
- Angiodysplasia
  - Vascular malformations of GI tract
  - Prone to bleeding
  - Commonly occur in aortic stenosis patients
- Deficiency of von Willebrand factor
  - High shearing force caused by aortic stenosis
  - Uncoiling of vWF multimers
  - Exposes cleavage site for ADAMST13
- Improves after aortic valve surgery

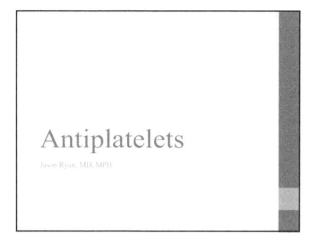

Antiplatelets

Jason Ryan, MD, MPH

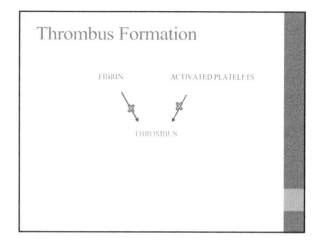

Thrombus Formation

FIBRIN   ACTIVATED PLATELETS

THROMBUS

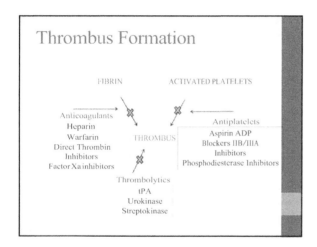

Thrombus Formation

FIBRIN   ACTIVATED PLATELETS

Anticoagulants
Heparin
Warfarin   THROMBUS
Direct Thrombin
Inhibitors
Factor Xa inhibitors

Antiplatelets
Aspirin ADP
Blockers IIB/IIIA
Inhibitors
Phosphodiesterase Inhibitors

Thrombolytics
tPA
Urokinase
Streptokinase

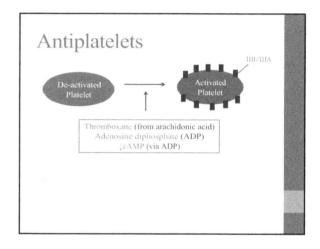

Antiplatelets

IIB/IIIA

De-activated Platelet → Activated Platelet

Thromboxane (from arachidonic acid)
Adenosine diphosphate (ADP)
↓cAMP (via ADP)

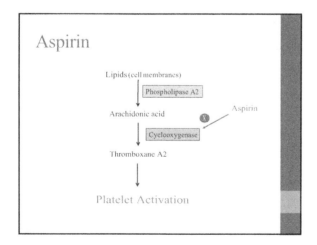

Aspirin

Lipids (cell membranes)

Phospholipase A2

Arachidonic acid   Aspirin

Cyclooygenase

Thromboxane A2

Platelet Activation

Aspirin

- Inhibits COX-1 and COX-2
  - Both found in platelets
- Blunts conversion of AA to TXA2
- ↓ platelet activity
- Also inhibits production of prostaglandins

30

Eicosanoids

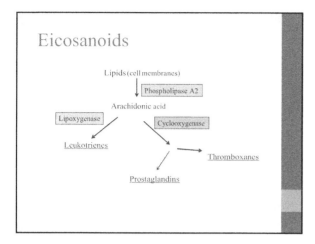

Lipids (cell membranes)

→ Phospholipase A2

Arachidonic acid

Lipoxygenase   Cyclooxygenase

Leukotrienes   Thromboxanes

Prostaglandins

Eicosanoids

Mediator	Effects
PGE$_2$	Redness (vasodilation) Edema (permeability) Fever (hypothalamus) Pain (nerves) Renal vasodilation (afferent)
PGE$_2$/PGI$_2$	Protect GI mucosa
TXA$_2$	Platelet activation

Ricciotti E, FitzGerald G; Prostaglandins and Inflammation
Arterioscler Thromb Vasc Biol. 2011 May; 31(5): 986–1000.

NSAIDs
Ibuprofen, naproxen, indomethacin, ketorolac, diclofenac

- Aspirin is technically NSAID
- NSAIDS reversibly inhibit COX-1 and COX-2
- Aspirin irreversibly inhibits COX-1 and COX-2
- Decreases activity for lifetime of platelet (7-10 days)
- All NSAIDs may cause bleeding
- All NSAIDs reduce pain, inflammation via ↓ PGs

Aspirin
Common antiplatelet uses

- Coronary disease
  - Acute myocardial infarction/unstable angina
  - Secondary prevention
- Stroke
  - Acute ischemic stroke
  - Secondary prevention

Aspirin
Adverse Effects

- Bleeding
- Gastritis/Ulcers
  - COX important for maintenance of GI mucosa
- Tinnitus
  - Caused by salicylate (aspirin metabolite: salicylic acid)
  - Alters cochlear nerve function
  - Rare: Usually occurs with very high doses
  - Resolves with discontinuation

Aspirin
Adverse Effects

- Reye's syndrome
  - Liver failure and encephalopathy
  - Associated with aspirin use in children
  - Aspirin not generally used in kids (exception: Kawasaki)

Thienopyridines
Ticlopidine, clopidogrel, prasugrel

Ticlopidine

- Irreversible $P2Y_{12}$ receptor blockers
- Block effects of ADP on platelets
- Used in aspirin allergy
- Added to aspirin for prevention of MI, Stroke
- Major adverse effect is bleeding
- Rare, dangerous adverse effect: TTP

TTP
Thrombotic Thrombocytopenic Purpura

- Associated with thienopyridine drugs
- Severe thrombocytopenia
- Microangiopathic hemolytic anemia
- Neurologic abnormalities
- Deficient activity of ADAMTS13
- Antibodies to ADAMTS13

Ticagrelor

- Cyclo-pentyl-triazolo-pyrimidine (CPTP)
  - NOT a thienopyridine
- Reversible antagonist to $P2Y_{12}$ receptor
- Unique side effect: Dyspnea
  - Mechanism unclear

Phosphodiesterase Inhibitors
PDE Inhibitors

- Inhibit phosphodiesterase III in platelets
- PDE breaksdown cAMP
- ↑ cAMP □ ↓ platelet activation
- Two drugs in class: dipyridamole, cilostazol

Dipyridamole

- PDEIII inhibitor
- Inhibits platelet activation
- Also blocks adenosine uptake by cells
  - Adenosine = vasodilator
  - Raises adenosine levels □ vasodilation
- Used with aspirin for stroke prevention (antiplatelet)
- Used in chemical cardiac stress testing (vasodilator)

Cilostazol

- PDEIII inhibitor
- Inhibits platelet activation
- Also raises cAMP in vascular smooth muscle
- Vasodilator
- Rarely used for anti-platelet effects
- Used in peripheral arterial disease

Phosphodiesterase Inhibitors
Dipyridamole, Cilostazol

- Many side effects related to vasodilation
  - Headache
  - Flushing
  - Hypotension

IIB/IIIA Receptor Blockers

- Abciximab, eptifibatide, tirofiban
- Bind and block IIB/IIIA receptors
- Abciximab: Fab fragment of antibody to IIB/IIIA
- IV drugs used in acute coronary syndromes/stenting

Eptifibatide   Tirofiban

IIB/IIIA Receptor Blockers

- Main adverse effect is bleeding
- Can cause thrombocytopenia
  - May occur within hours of administration
  - Mechanism poorly understood
  - Must monitor platelet count after administration

Antiplatelet Drugs

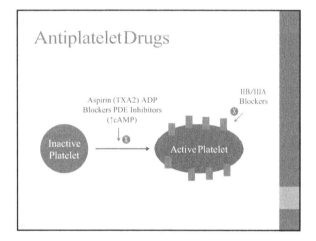

Aspirin (TXA2) ADP
Blockers PDE Inhibitors
(↑cAMP)

IIB/IIIA
Blockers

Inactive Platelet → Active Platelet

Anticoagulant Drugs

Jason Ryan, MD, MPH

Thrombus Disorders

Disease	→	Thrombus Location
Atrial Fibrillation		Left atrial appendage
Myocardial Infarction		Coronary artery
DVT/PE		Deep vein/pulm artery
Critical Limb Ischemia		Peripheral circulation

Antithrombotic Drugs

- Acute therapy: Help eliminate clot already formed
- Prevention: Lower risk of clot in high risk patients

Thrombus Formation

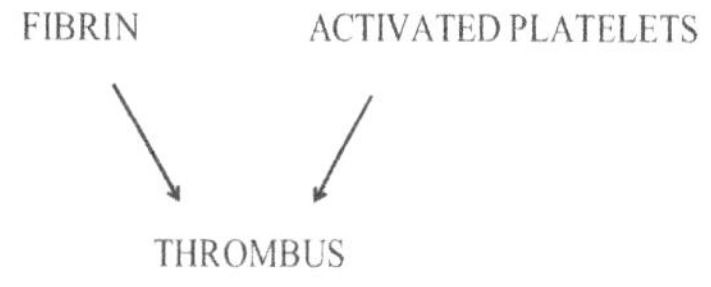

FIBRIN   ACTIVATED PLATELETS

THROMBUS

Blood thinners

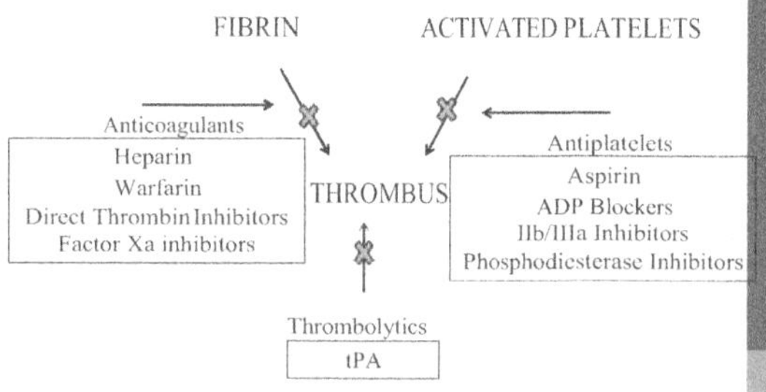

FIBRIN   ACTIVATED PLATELETS

Anticoagulants
Heparin
Warfarin
Direct Thrombin Inhibitors
Factor Xa inhibitors

THROMBUS

Antiplatelets
Aspirin
ADP Blockers
IIb/IIIa Inhibitors
Phosphodiesterase Inhibitors

Thrombolytics
tPA

Bleeding

- Thrombus formation very beneficial
- Prevents/stops bleeding
- BLEEDING: common side effect
- Can occur with all antithrombotic/antiplatelet drugs

Clotting versus Bleeding

Myocardial Infarction
Pulmonary Embolism
Deep VeinThrombosis
Stoke

GI Bleeding
CNS Bleeding
Bruising

Coagulation Cascade

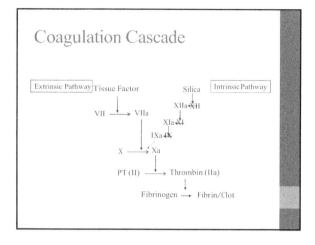

PTT
Activated Partial Thromboplastin Time

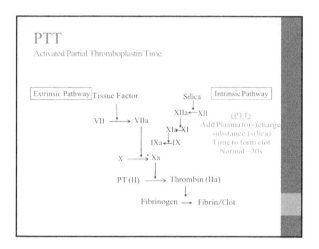

PT
Prothrombin Time

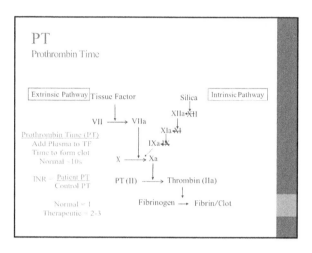

Thrombin Time

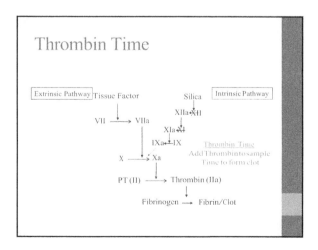

Heparin

- Polymer (glycosaminoglycan)
- Occurs naturally (found in mast cells)
- Molecules with varying chain lengths
- Used in two forms:
  - Unfractionated: widely varying polymer chain lengths
  - Low molecular weight: Smaller polymers only

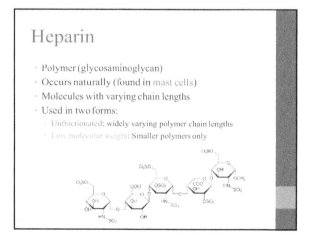

Unfractionated Heparin

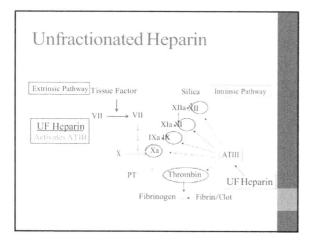

Extrinsic Pathway | Tissue Factor   Silica   Intrinsic Pathway

UF Heparin
Activates ATIII

VII → VII

XIIa→XII

XIa→XI

IXa→IX

X   Xa

ATIII

PT   Thrombin   UF Heparin

Fibrinogen → Fibrin/Clot

Unfractionated Heparin (UFH)

- Given IV or SQ ☐ acute onset
- Increases PTT
  - Effects many components of intrinsic pathway
  - HeparIN = INtrinsic (PTT)
- Will also increase thrombin time
- Can increase PT at high dosages
- Lots of binding to plasma proteins, cells
  - Highly variable response from patient to patient
  - Dose must be adjusted to reach goal PTT

Protamine

- Reversal agent for unfractionated heparin
  - Less effective with LMWH
- Binds heparin ☐ neutralizes drug
- Used in heparin overdose
- Used in cardiac surgery
  - High dose heparin administered for heart-lung bypass
  - Quick reversal at completion of case

Unfractionated Heparin (UFH)

- Uses:
  - Acute management: DVT/PE, MI, Stroke
  - Prophylaxis for DVT in hospitalized patients (SQ)

Unfractionated Heparin (UFH)

- Side Effects
  - Mainly bleeding and thrombocytopenia
  - Osteoporosis (long term use)
  - Elevated AST/ALT (mild)

Heparin and Thrombocytopenia

- Many patients ☐ mild (10-20%) ↓ platelets
  - "Non-immune" thrombocytopenia
  - Direct suppressive effect platelet production
- Heparin-induced thrombocytopenia (HIT)
  - Immune-mediated reaction
  - Immune complexes bind platelet factor4-heparin
  - Type II hypersensitivity reaction

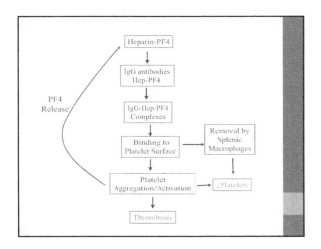

HIT
Heparin-induced thrombocytopenia

- 5-10 days after exposure to heparin
- Abrupt fall in platelets (>50%)
- Arterial/vein thrombosis
- Rare: 0.2 – 5% Heparin patients
- Patients with HIT must use alternative drugs
    - Lepirudin, Bivalirudin (direct thrombin inhibitors)

HIT
Heparin-induced thrombocytopenia

- Presumptive diagnosis:
    - Significant drop in platelet count
    - Thrombosis formation
- Definitive diagnosis: HIT antibody testing
    - Autoantibodies to platelet factor 4 complexed with heparin

Low Molecular Weight Heparin
Enoxaparin

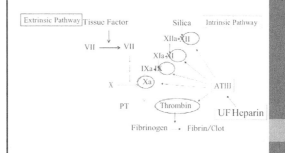

Low Molecular Weight Heparin
Enoxaparin

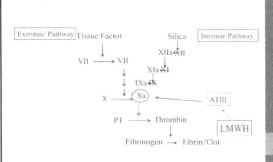

Low Molecular Weight Heparin
Enoxaparin

- Dose based on weight – no titrating
    - Reduced binding to plasma proteins and cells
- Given SQ
- Lower incidence of HIT (but may still cause!)

Low Molecular Weight Heparin
Enoxaparin

- Will not affect thrombin time (like UF heparin)
- PTT not sensitive to LMWH-induced changes
  - Unlike UF heparin, only factor X effected

UFH

PTT

LMWH

Plasma Concentration

Low Molecular Weight Heparin
Enoxaparin

- If monitoring required, must check anti Xa levels
  - Limited/insensitive affect on PTT
  - Standard dose based on weight
  - Usually no monitoring used
  - Exceptions: Obesity and renal failure

Anti-Xa Level

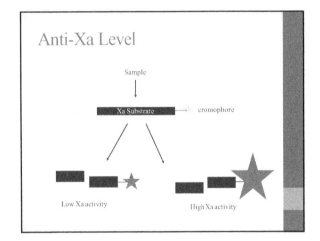

Sample

Xa Substrate ---> cromophore

Low Xa activity

High Xa activity

Factor Xa Inhibitors

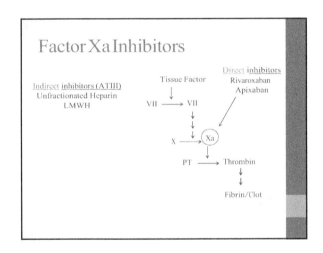

Indirect inhibitors (ATIII)
Unfractionated Heparin
LMWH

Tissue Factor

Direct inhibitors
Rivaroxaban
Apixaban

VII ---> VII

X ---> Xa

PT ---> Thrombin

Fibrin/Clot

Factor Xa Inhibitors

- Rivaroxaban, Apixaban
- Used in atrial fibrillation as alternatives to warfarin
  - Do not require monitoring of PT/INR
  - Standard dosing
- Can increase PT and PTT (Xa in both pathways)
- Will not affect thrombin time

Direct Thrombin Inhibitors

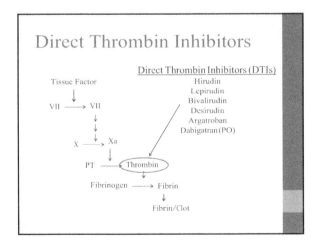

Direct Thrombin Inhibitors (DTIs)
Hirudin
Lepirudin
Bivalirudin
Desirudin
Argatroban
Dabigatran (PO)

Tissue Factor

VII ---> VII

X ---> Xa

PT ---> Thrombin

Fibrinogen ---> Fibrin

Fibrin/Clot

38

Direct Thrombin Inhibitors
Uses

- Can prolong PT, PTT, and thrombin time
- Thrombin activity common to all tests
- Only UF heparin and DTIs prolong thrombin time
  - Requires an inhibitor of thrombin function
  - UF Heparin: ATIII
  - DTIs: Direct drug effect

Direct Thrombin Inhibitors
Uses

- Patients with HIT
  - Hirudin, lepirudin, bivalirudin, desirudin, argatroban
  - Stop heparin, start DTI
  - PTT often monitored
- Acute coronary syndromes, coronary interventions
  - Bivalirudin
- Atrial fibrillation
  - Dabigatran (oral)
  - Standard dosing: does not require PT/INR monitoring

Warfarin

- Vitamin K Factors: II, VII, IX, and X
- Warfarin: Antagonist to vitamin K
- ↓ levels of all vitamin K dependent factors

Vitamin K

- Forms γ-carboxyglutamate (Gla) residues

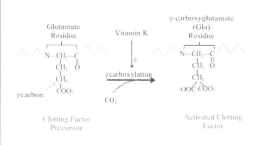

Vitamin K

- Found in green, leafy vegetables (K1 form)
  - Cabbage, kale, spinach
  - Also egg yolk, liver
- Also synthesized by GI bacteria (K2 form)

Warfarin
Vitamin K Antagonist

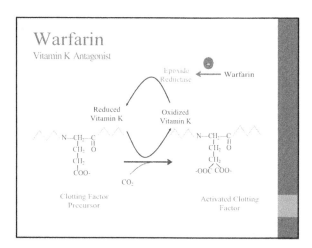

Warfarin

- Takes days to achieve its effects
  - Time required for clotting factor levels to fall
- Dose adjusted to reach target PT/INR
  - Drugs effect varies with diet (vitamin K)
  - Antibiotics may ↓ GI bacteria □ ↓ vitamin K □ ↑ INR
  - Some drugs interfere with metabolism

Vitamin K Dependent Factors

| Extrinsic Pathway | Tissue Factor | | Silica | Intrinsic Pathway |

VII —— VII
XIIa→XII
XIa→XI
IXa→IX
X ··· Xa
PT ··· Thrombin
Fibrinogen —→ Fibrin/Clot

Vitamin K Dependent Factors

- Factor VII has shortest half life
  - First level to fall after Warfarin administration
- Only PT captures factor VII activity
- PTT less sensitive to Warfarin
- Thrombin time normal

Protein	Half-life (hours)
Factor VII	4-6
Protein C	8-10
Factor X	24-40
Protein S	40-60
Prothrombin (II)	60-72

Warfarin
Prothrombotic Effects

- Protein C: anti-clotting factor with short half-life
- Also vitamin K dependent
- Initial warfarin Rx □ protein C deficient
  - This is pro-thrombotic
  - Brief...eventually other factors fall □ antithrombotic

Protein	Half-life (hours)
Factor VII	4 - 6
Protein C	8 - 10
Factor X	24 - 40
Protein S	40 - 60
Prothrombin (II)	60 - 72

Warfarin
Prothrombotic Effects

- Should you start another drug (heparin) anytime you start warfarin?
  - Yes, but this is usually not an issue
  - For clot disorders (DVT/PE) heparin used for acute onset
  - Heparin □ anticoagulation during initial warfarin therapy
- One exception: Atrial fibrillation
  - No active clot; just risk of clot
  - Often start warfarin without heparin
  - Brief increase in risk of clot is very low

Warfarin
Adverse Effects

- Crosses placenta
  - Avoided in pregnancy
  - Fetal warfarin syndrome: abnormal fetal development
  - Unfractionated heparin often used (does not cross)
- Side Effects:
  - Mainly bleeding
  - Skin necrosis

Warfarin Skin Necrosis

- Rare complication of therapy
- Occurs in patients with protein C deficiency
- Can also occur with very high dosages
- Initial exposure to warfarin □ ↓ protein C
- Result: thrombosis of skin tissue
- Large dark, purple skin lesions

Warfarin
Uses

- Stroke prevention atrial fibrillation
- Mechanical heart valves
- DVT/PE

Chronic Oral Anticoagulation

- Several Indications
  - Atrial Fibrillation
  - Mechanical heart valve
  - Prior DVT or PE
- Prior Standard: Warfarin
  - Oral drug, Low Cost
  - Downside: Requires INR checks (monthly blood draw)

Novel Oral Anticoagulants (NOACs)
Alternatives to Warfarin

- Factor Xa inhibitors
  - #1: Rivaroxaban
  - #2: Apixaban
- Direct Thrombin inhibitors
  - #3: Dabigatran
- Upside: No INR checks…consistent dose
- Downsides
  - Cost $$
  - Reversal agents - Idarucizumab

Thrombolysis

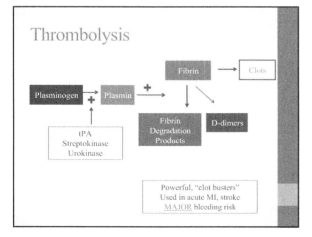

Plasminogen → Plasmin + → Fibrin → Clots

tPA
Streptokinase
Urokinase

Fibrin Degradation Products

D-dimers

Powerful, "clot busters"
Used in acute MI, stroke
MAJOR bleeding risk

Reversal of drugs

- Fresh Frozen Plasma (FFP)
  - Plasma after removal of RBC, WBC, and Plt
  - Frozen for storage
  - Once thawed, must be used within 24hrs
  - Clotting factors degrade
  - Corrects deficiencies of any clotting factor
  - PT/PTT will normalize after infusion

Reversal of drugs

- Vitamin K
  - Reverses warfarin
  - Used with ↑ INR in absence of serious bleeding
  - Given PO or IV
  - IV can cause anaphylaxis
- INR 3-5: Hold warfarin
- INR 5-9: Hold warfarin, Oral vitamin K
- INR >9: Consider IV vitamin K, FFP

Severe bleeding + ↑INR = administer FFP

Hemolysis Basics

Jason Ryan, MD, MPH

Hemolysis

- Destruction of red blood cells
- Causes a normocytic anemia

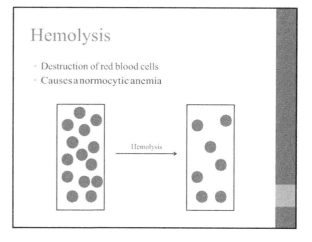

Normocytic Anemias

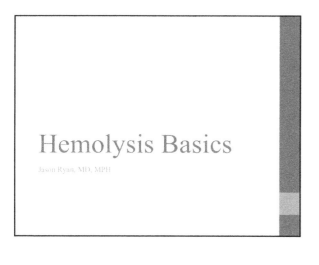

Hemolysis
Extrinsic versus Intrinsic

- Extrinsic cause
  - Cause is extrinsic to the red cell
  - Antibodies
  - Mechanical trauma (narrow vessels)
  - RBC infection
- Intrinsic cause
  - Cause is intrinsic to red blood cells
  - Failure of membrane, hemoglobin, or enzymes
  - Membrane: Hereditary spherocytosis
  - Enzyme: G6PD deficiency
  - Hemoglobin: Sickle cell anemia (Abnormal Hgb)

Normocytic Anemias

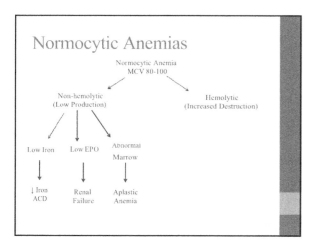

Hemolysis
Consequences

- Normocytic anemia
- Elevated plasma LDH
  - Lactate dehydrogenase
  - Glycolysis enzyme
  - Converts pyruvate → lactate
  - Spills out of RBCs

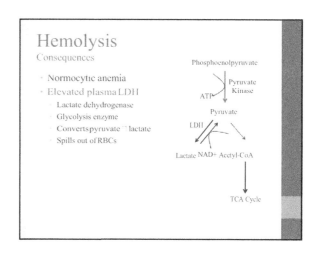

Reticulocytes

- Immature red blood cells
- Usually about 1-2% of RBCs in peripheral blood
- Increased reticulocyte count: Hallmark of hemolysis

Hemolysis

↓

↑ EPO

↓

↑ Reticulocyte

Reticulocyte Count

- ↑ reticulocytes: normal marrow response to anemia
- Key blood test in normocytic anemias
- Normocytic anemia: ↓ production or ↑ destruction
- Reticulocyte count differentiates between causes
  - Low retic count: Underproduction
  - High retic count: Increased destruction (hemolysis)

Reticulocyte Count

- Normal: 1 to 2 %
- Anemia: 4-5%
- Must be corrected for degree of anemia
- If <2% ☐ inadequate bone marrow response

Hct 45 (normal) ⟶ Hct 11
Retic 1% (normal)   Retic 8%

Corrected RC = 8% * (11/45) = 2%

Reticulocyte Production Index

- Normal reticulocytes circulate ~1day
- In anemia ☐ premature release of reticulocytes
- Can live longer ☐ circulate longer
- RPI corrects for longer life of reticulocytes in anemia
- RPI < 2% seen with bone marrow failure

$$RPI = \frac{\text{Corrected Retic \%}}{\text{Maturation Time}}$$

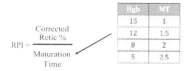

Hgb	MT
15	1
12	1.5
8	2
5	2.5

Hemolysis
Consequences

- Elevated unconjugated (indirect) bilirubin
- Not water soluble
- Bound to albumin in plasma

Heme ⟶ Bilirubin

Jaundice

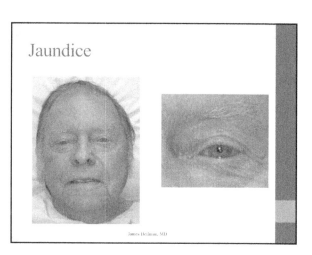

James Heilman, MD

Gallstones

- ↑ risk in hemolysis
- Pigment stones
  - Contain bilirubin
  - Less common type of gallstone (more common: cholesterol)

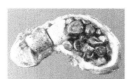

Emmanuelm/Wikipedia

Hemolysis
Intravascular versus Extravascular

- Intravascular hemolysis
  - Occurs inside blood vessels
- Extravascular hemolysis
  - Occurs in liver and spleen
- Both cause normocytic anemia and ↑ retic count

Extravascular Hemolysis

- Liver
  - Receives large portion cardiac output
  - Can remove severely damaged RBCs
- Spleen
  - Destroys poorly deformable RBCs
  - Cords of Billroth: Vascular channels that end blindly
  - Found in red pulp of spleen
  - RBCs must deform to pass through slits in walls of cords
  - Old ("senescent") or damaged RBCs remain in the cords
  - Phagocytosed by the macrophages
  - Hemolysis disorders □ ↑ splenic removal of RBCs

Spleen

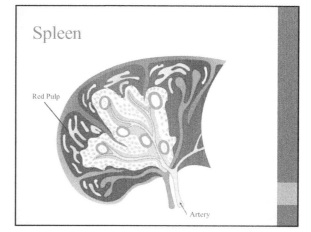

Red Pulp

Artery

Intravascular Hemolysis

- Destruction of RBCs inside blood vessels
  - Outside of spleen
- Mechanical trauma
  - Narrowed vessels
  - Small vessels: thrombus ("microangiopathic")
  - Large vessels: mechanical heart valves

Haptoglobin

- Plasma protein
- Binds free hemoglobin
- Haptoglobin-hemoglobin complex removed by liver
- ↓ serum haptoglobin with hemolysis

Haptoglobin

- Intravascular: Hgb released directly into plasma
  - Haptoglobin very low or undetectable
- Extravascular: Some Hgb released from spleen
  - Haptoglobin can be low or normal
- Classically taught as low in intravascular only
- Studies show can be low in both types

Kormoczi G. Influence of clinical factors on the haemolysis marker haptoglobin. Eur J Clin Invest 2006 Mar;36(3)

Haptoglobin

- Produced by the liver
- Acute phase reactant
- Increased levels with inflammation
- Decreased levels in cirrhosis

Hemolyisis
Urine findings

- No bilirubin
  - Unconjugated bilirubin not water soluble
  - Cannot pass into urine

Hemolyisis
Urine findings

- Intravascular hemolyisis
  - Haptoglobin saturation ☐ free excess hemoglobin
  - "Hemoglobinemia"
  - Filtered in kidneys ☐ hemoglobinuria
  - Some reabsorbed in proximal tubules
  - Iron converted into ferritin ☐ hemosiderin in tubular cells
  - Tubular cells slough into urine
  - Prussian blue stain on sediment shows hemosiderinuria

Hemolyisis
Urine findings

- Hemoglobin part of urine dipstick
- Hgb may turn urine red/brown
  - Also occurs in rhabdomyolysis
  - Myoglobin from muscle damage
- No red cells plus + Hgb

Urine test strip

Leukocytes
Nitrite
Urobilinogen
Protein
pH
Haemoglobin
Specific gravity
Ketone
Bilirubin
Glucose

James Heilman, MD -

Hemolysis
Classic Findings

- Normocytic anemia
- ↑ LDH
- ↑ Indirect bilirubin
- ↑ Reticulocyte count
- ↓ Haptoglobin (lower in intravascular)
- Urine Hgb and hemosiderin (intravascular)

Parvovirus B19

- DNA virus
- Replicates in RBC progenitor cells
- ↓erythropoiesis

Parvovirus B19

- Healthy patients:
  - RBC production returns 10 to 14 days; mild/no anemia
- Hemolysis patients
  - Increased RBC turnover
  - Lack of erythropoiesis leads to severe anemia
  - Pallor, weakness, and lethargy

Parvovirus B19

- "Aplastic Crisis" in patients with chronic hemolysis
  - Sickle cell anemia
  - Hereditary spherocytosis
  - Beta thalassemia major
- Classic scenario:
  - Worsening anemia with LOW reticulocyte count

Back and Abdominal Pain

- Seen in some hemolytic syndromes
- Abdominal pain can be caused by splenomegaly
- May be due to smooth muscle spasm
- Nitric oxide: scavenged by free hemoglobin
- Common in some hemolytic disorders
  - Paroxysmal nocturnal hemoglobinuria
  - G6PD deficiency

Extrinsic Hemolysis

Jason Ryan, MD, MPH

Normocytic Anemias

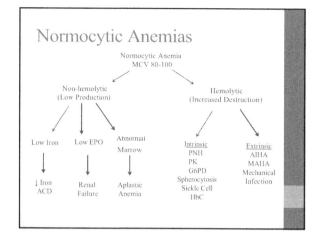

Normocytic Anemia
MCV 80-100

Non-hemolytic (Low Production)

Hemolytic (Increased Destruction)

Low Iron | Low EPO | Abnormal Marrow

↓ Iron ACD | Renal Failure | Aplastic Anemia

Intrinsic
PNH
PK
G6PD
Spherocytosis
Sickle Cell
HbC

Extrinsic
AIHA
MAHA
Mechanical
Infection

Extrinsic Hemolysis

- Antibodies
- Trauma/shearing
- Red cell infections

AIHA
Autoimmune Hemolytic Anemia

- Red cell destruction from autoantibodies
- Results in extravascular hemolysis
- Red cell membrane removed in pieces by spleen
- Can be "warm" or "cold"

Warm AIHA

- Most common type of AIHA
- Antibodies bind at body temp 37°C ("warm")
- IgG antibodies against RBC surface antigens

Warm AIHA
Signs and symptoms

- Anemia
  - Fatigue
  - Pallor (pale skin)
  - Dyspnea
  - Tachycardia
- Extravascular hemolysis
  - Jaundice
  - Splenomegaly

Warm AIHA
Diagnostic Findings

- Spherocytes
  - Smaller than normal RBCs
  - Spherical

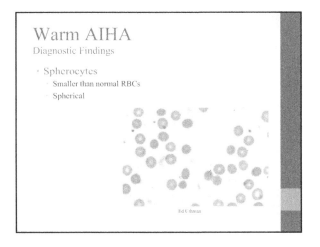

Ed Uthman

Direct Antiglobulin Test
DAT or Coombs Test

- Test for red blood cell antibodies
- Patient RBCs plus anti IgG antiserum
- Positive if agglutination occurs
- Indicates patient's RBCs covered with IgG

Direct Antiglobulin Test
DAT or Coombs Test

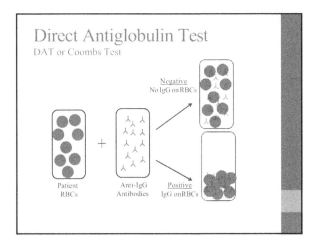

Indirect Antiglobulin Test
Indirect Coombs

- Also a test for red blood cell antibodies
- Not generally used in warm/cold AIHA
- Tests for antibodies in the serum
- Patient's serum (not RBCs) tested
- Added to RBCs
- Indicates antibodies to RBC components

Indirect Antiglobulin Test
Indirect Coombs

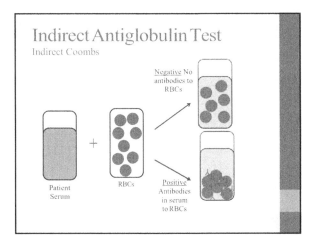

Antiglobulin Tests

- Direct antiglobulin test
  - Test for antibodies bound to RBC's
  - Commonly used in hemolytic anemias
- Indirect antiglobulin test
  - Test for antibodies in serum
  - Will serum react with RBCs?

Warm AIHA
Associated Conditions

- Most cases idiopathic
- Associated with:
  - Lupus
  - Non-Hodgkin lymphoma
  - Chronic lymphocytic leukemia (CLL)

Methyldopa
α methyldopa

- Antihypertensive drug of choice in pregnancy
  - Agonists to CNS α2 receptors
  - Synapses believe too much sympathetic outflow
  - Decrease sympathetic tone in body
- Associated with warm AIHA

Øyvind Holmstad/Wikipedia

Methyldopa
α methyldopa

- Triggers production of RBC antibodies
  - Unclear mechanism
  - Drug may alter Rh antigens on red cells
  - Red cells bind antibody in absence of drug
- Direct Coombs test: positive

Penicillin

- High doses can lead to hemolytic anemia
- PCN binds to surface RBCs ("hapten")
  - Elicits immune response only when bound
- Antibodies against PCN bound to RBCs
- Direct Coombs test: positive

Warm AIHA
Treatment

- Glucocorticoids
- Immunosuppressants
- Splenectomy

Cold AIHA

- Less common type of AIHA
- Antibodies bind at <30°C ("cold")
  - Occurs in limbs
  - Also fingertips, toes, nose, ears
- May present with painful fingers/toes
  - Purple discoloration
- Symptoms associated with cold exposure

Cold AIHA
Cold Agglutinin Disease

- Caused by IgM antibodies that agglutinate RBCs
- RBCs warmed in central organs ☐ IgM lost
- Leaves bound C3 on RBCs
- DAT positive only for C3

Martin Brändli /Wikipedia

Direct Antiglobulin Test
DAT or Coombs Test

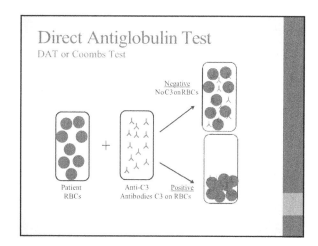

Patient RBCs   Anti-C3 Antibodies

Negative
No C3 on RBCs

Positive
C3 on RBCs

Cold AIHA
Cold Agglutinin Disease

- Usually causes extravascular hemolyisis
  - C3 coated RBCs removed by spleen
  - Often engulfed whole
  - Spherocytosis less common than in warm AIHA
- Intravascular hemolysis rarely occurs
  - Complement usually does not activate
  - RBCs: complement inhibitory molecules (CD55/CD59)
  - Complement must be significantly activated to lyse cells

Cold AIHA
Associated conditions

- Can be seen in chronic lymphocytic leukemia (CLL)
- Often occurs secondary to infection
  - Mycoplasma pneumonia
  - Epstein–Barr virus (Infectious mononucleosis)

Cold AIHA
Treatment

- Avoid cold (stay warm!)
- Immunosuppressants

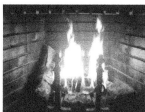

Public Domain/Wikipedia

MAHA
Microangiopathic hemolytic anemia

- Shearing of RBCs in small blood vessels
- Thrombi in microvasculature ☐ narrowing
- Blood smear: schistocytes
- Seen in:
  - TTP
  - HUS
  - DIC

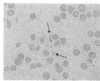

Paulo Henrique Orlandi Mourao

Malignant Hypertension

- Associated with MAHA
- Endothelial injury ☐ thrombus formation
- Improved with BP control

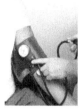

Public Domain

Mechanical Hemolysis

- Shear forces destroy RBCs in large blood vessels
- Seen in:
  - Aortic stenosis
  - Mechanical heart valves
  - Left ventricular assist devices
- Hemolytic anemia may occur
- Schistocytes can be seen on blood smear

Red Blood Cell Infections

- May cause hemolytic anemia
- Classic infectious agents: Malaria, Babesia

Babesia
Ring Forms

Malaria
Trophozoite Ring

CDC/Public Domain

Intrinsic Hemolysis

Jason Ryan, MD, MPH

Normocytic Anemias

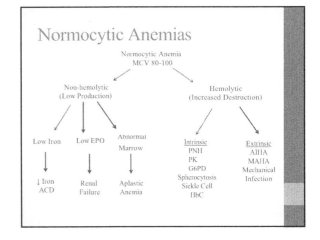

Normocytic Anemia
MCV 80-100

Non-hemolytic
(Low Production)

Hemolytic
(Increased Destruction)

Low Iron   Low EPO   Abnormal
Marrow

Intrinsic
PNH
PK
G6PD
Spherocytosis
Sickle Cell
HbC

Extrinsic
AIHA
MAHA
Mechanical
Infection

↓ Iron
ACD

Renal
Failure

Aplastic
Anemia

PNH
Paroxysmal Nocturnal Hemoglobinuria

- RBC destruction via complement system
- Loss of protective proteins in RBC membrane
  - Decay Accelerating Factor (DAF/CD55)
  - MAC inhibitory protein (CD59)
- Predominantly intravascular hemolysis
- Some extravascular hemolysis
  - Macrophage destruction of RBCs opsonized with C3 fragments

PNH
Paroxysmal Nocturnal Hemoglobinuria

- Acquired genetic mutation in stem cell
  - Loss of glycosylphosphatidylinositol (GPI) anchor
  - Attaches proteins to cell surface
  - Lead to loss of DAF/CD59 on RBC cell membranes
- Platelets/WBCs may also have lysis

PNH
Paroxysmal Nocturnal Hemoglobinuria

- Classically causes sudden hemolysis at night
  - Slowing of respiratory rate with sleep
  - Also shallow breathing
  - Mild ↑CO_2 ⟶ mild resp. acidosis ⟶ ↑ complement activity
- Fatigue, dyspnea
  - Anemia from hemolysis
  - May also lose iron in urine
  - Iron-deficiency is common

PNH
Paroxysmal Nocturnal Hemoglobinuria

- Abdominal pain (smooth muscle tension)
- Thrombosis
  - Leading cause of death
  - Usually venous clots
  - Unusual locations: portal, mesenteric, cerebral veins
- Some patients develop acute myeloid leukemia (AML)
  - Stem cell mutation progresses to acute leukemia
  - Lifetime risk: 5 percent or less

PNH
Paroxysmal Nocturnal Hemoglobinuria

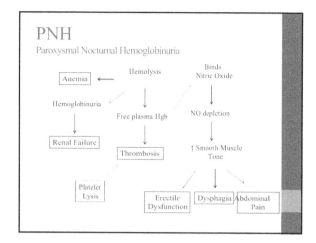

PNH
Diagnosis

- Suspected with hemolysis, unexplained thrombosis
- Labs may show evidence of hemolysis
  - LDH, Low haptoglobin
  - Urine hemoglobin or hemosiderin
- Direct antibody testing (Coombs) will be negative
- Flow cytometry confirms diagnosis
  - Monoclonal antibodies to GPI-anchored proteins
  - Cells will be deficient in GPI-anchored proteins

Eculizumab

- Anti-complement therapy
- Antibody that binds to complement component C5
  - Prevents cleavage to C5a and C5b
- Blocks formation of membrane attack complex (MAC)
- Protects against intravascular hemolysis
- Does not protect against extravascular hemolysis
  - C3 fragments still bind RBCs □ spleen
  - Treated patients may still have mild anemia
- Results in stable Hgb levels, fewer transfusions

Pyruvate Kinase Deficiency

- Deficiency of pyruvate kinase
- Key enzyme in glycolysis
- RBCs most effected
  - No mitochondria
  - Require PK for anaerobic metabolism
- Membrane failure □ phagocytosis in spleen

Phosphoenolpyruvate → Pyruvate Kinase → Pyruvate → Lactate / TCA Cycle

Pyruvate Kinase Deficiency

- Autosomal recessive disorder
- Usually presents as newborn
- Extravascular hemolysis
- Splenomegaly
- Disease severity ranges based on enzyme activity

G6PD Deficiency
Glucose-6-Phosphate Dehydrogenase

- Key enzyme in HMP shunt
- HMP shunt necessary for generation of NADPH
- NADPH protects RBCs from oxidative damage

G6PD Deficiency
Glucose-6-Phosphate Dehydrogenase

- H_2O_2 toxic to RBCs
- H_2O_2 generation triggered by:
  - Infections
  - Drugs
  - Fava beans
- Need NADPH to degrade H_2O_2
- Absence of required NADPH □ hemolysis

G6PD Deficiency
Glucose-6-Phosphate Dehydrogenase

- X-linked recessive disorder (males)
- Most common human enzyme disorder
- Recurrent hemolysis after exposure to trigger
  - Red cells become rigid
  - Consumed by splenic macrophages (extravascular)
  - Some lysis in blood vessels (intravascular)

Exposure
to   ⟶   Hemolysis
Trigger

G6PD Deficiency
Triggers

- Infection: Macrophages generate free radicals
- Fava beans: Contain oxidants
- Drugs:
  - Antibiotics (sulfa drugs, dapsone, nitrofurantoin, INH)
  - Anti-malarials (primaquine, quinidine)
  - Aspirin, acetaminophen (rare)

G6PD Deficiency
Glucose-6-Phosphate Dehydrogenase

- High prevalence in Africa, Asia, the Mediterranean
  - May protect against malaria

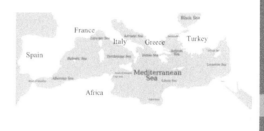

G6PD Deficiency
Classic presentation

- Patient from Africa, Asia, Mediterranean
- Jaundice, dark urine, anemia
- May have back pain (free Hgb)
- Onset after exposure to trigger

G6PD Deficiency
Glucose-6-Phosphate Dehydrogenase

- Classic findings: Heinz bodies and bite cells
- Heinz bodies: oxidized Hgb precipitated in RBCs
  - Seen with Heinz body stain ("Heinz body preparation")
- Bite cells: phagocytic removal by splenic macrophages

Heinz bodies   Bite cells

G6PD Deficiency
Diagnosis and Treatment

- Diagnosis:
  - Fluorescent spot test
  - Detects generation of NADPH from NADP
  - Add glucose-6-phosphate and NADP to red cells
  - Positive test if blood spot fails to fluoresce under UV light
- Must test outside of acute attack
  - Triggers □ destruction of enzyme-poor cells
  - Remaining cells may have normal enzyme levels
- Treatment:
  - Avoidance of triggers

Hereditary Spherocytosis

- Hereditary disorder
  - Can be autosomal dominant or recessive
- Results in spherocytes
  - Slightly smaller than normal RBCs
  - Spherical shape
  - Lacks central pallor

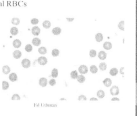

Ed Uthman

Hereditary Spherocytosis

- Cytoskeleton abnormality
  - Abnormal proteins that tie cytoskeleton to RBC membrane
  - Common involves spectrin
  - Other proteins: ankyrin, band 3, band 4.2

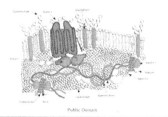

Public Domain

Hereditary Spherocytosis

- O2 carrying function of spherocytes normal
- Disease from chronic destruction in spleen
  - Splenomegaly (growth of splenic macrophages)
  - Increased bilirubin
  - Jaundice
  - Bilirubin gallstones

Hereditary Spherocytosis

- Progressive loss of cell membrane
- Over time, more and more membrane lost
- Results in a high RDW

Number of cells — Normal / Spherocytosis

Hereditary Spherocytosis

- Volume does not change over time
- Results in a high MCHC
- MCV usually normal or low
  - Spherocytes: low MCV
  - Reticulocytes: high MCV

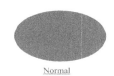

Normal   Same Vol. Smaller Cell ↑MCHC

Spherocyte

Hereditary Spherocytosis

- Loss of membrane flexibility ▯ more rigid cells
- High resistance to blood flow in small vessels

$$R = \frac{\Delta P}{Q} = \frac{8\,\eta\,(\text{viscosity})\,L\,(\text{length})}{\Pi\,r\,(\text{radius})^{4}}$$

Poiseuille's Law

Hereditary Spherocytosis

- Risk of aplastic crisis with parvovirus B19 infection
  - Patients dependent on marrow to replace hemolyzed cells
- Initial presentation may be a child with infection
  - Hemolysis compensated until B19 exposure
  - Spherocytosis seen on blood smear
  - Don't confuse with G6PD

Hereditary Spherocytosis
Diagnosis

- Osmotic fragility test
- Spherocytes: susceptible to osmotic lysis
  - Poor ability to swell like normal RBCs
  - Will lyse in hypotonic solution
- Measure Hgb release in hypotonic solution
- Osmotic fragility will be ↑ if spherocytosis present

Hereditary Spherocytosis

- Treatment: Splenectomy
- Spherocytes will persist but hemolysis resolves
- Howell–Jolly bodies appear
  - Some RBCs leave marrow with nuclear remnants
  - Normally cleared by spleen
  - Presence in peripheral blood indicates splenic dysfunction
- Classic finding: spherocytes and Howell-Jolly bodies
  - Indicates patient post-splenectomy for spherocytosis

Howell-Jolly Bodies

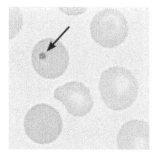

Paulo Henrique Orlandi Mourao/Mikael Häggström

Microcytic Anemias

Jason Ryan, MD, MPH

Red Blood Cell Measurements

- RBC count
  - Part of CBC with white cell count and platelets
- Hemoglobin
  - Concentration in g/dl
- Hematocrit
  - Volume % of red cells

Plasma

Leukocytes & thrombocytes

Formed elements

Erythrocytes

MesserWoland Wikipedia

Rule of 3

- Hgb = 3 x Red Blood Cell Count
- Hct = 3 x Hgb

Normal Values RBC
= 5 million cells/ul Hgb
= 15g/dl Hct = 45%

RBC Indices

- Measured by automated blood counters
- Measures of mean characteristics of RBCs
- Used in evaluation of anemias

RBC Indices

- Mean corpuscular volume (MCV)
  - Normal range: 80 to 100 femtoliters
- Mean corpuscular hemoglobin (MCH)
  - Amount (mass) of hemoglobin per red cell
  - Usually reported in picograms (per cell)
- Mean corpuscular Hgb concentration (MCHC)
  - Concentration of Hgb in red cells
  - Usually reported g/dL

Anemia Classification

- MCV commonly used to classify anemias

Microcytic MCV<80	Normocytic MCV 80-100	Macrocytic MCV>100
Iron deficiency	Iron deficiency	Folate/B12 deficiency
Anemia Chronic Disease	Anemia Chronic Disease	Orotic Aciduria
Thalassemia	Hemolysis	Liver disease
Lead poisoning	Aplastic anemia	Alcoholism
Sideroblastic Anemia	Kidney disease	Reticulocytosis

Microcytic Anemias

- Usually due to ↓ hemoglobin in red cells
- Usually associated with ↓ MCH and MCHC
- Low hemoglobin ☐ hypochromic RBCs on smear

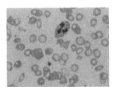

Roberto J. Galindo

Hemoglobin

- Globin chains
  - Proteins
  - 4 chains in 2 pairs
- Protoporphyrin
- Iron
- Microcytic anemia
  - Loss of iron
  - Loss of globins (thalassemia)
  - Loss of heme (lead, sideroblastic)

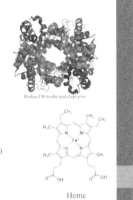

Richard Wheeler and Zephyris

Heme

Iron Absorption

- Heme iron
  - Found in meats
  - Easily absorbed
- Non-heme iron
  - Absorbed in Fe^{2+} state
  - Aided by vitamin C

Vitamin C

Fe^{3+} → Fe^{2+} Heme

Duodenal
Epithelial
Cell

Iron Metabolism

- Iron consumed in diet
- Uptake to plasma regulated by enterocytes
  - Iron transporter: ferroportin
  - Transports iron out of enterocytes and other cells
- Few mechanisms to excrete excess iron
  - Small amount in sweat, sloughing of skin/GI cells
  - Women lose iron from menstruation

Heme
Fe2+

Duodenal
Epithelial
Cell

FP   Fe2+

Iron Metabolism

- Iron always bound to a protein
- Transport protein: transferrin
  - Transported in blood via transferrin
  - ↑ transferrin when iron stores are low
- Storage protein: ferritin
  - Stored intracellularly as ferritin
  - Stored in macrophages of liver and bone

Clinical Iron Measurements

Test	Interpretation
Serum iron	Iron level
Total Iron Binding Capacity	Amount of transferrin in serum
Serum ferritin	Amount of storage iron
% saturation	Amount of transferrin bound to Fe

Iron Deficiency

- Lack of iron from gut
- Loss of iron (usually as blood)

Iron Deficiency
Inadequate GI uptake

- Babies
  - Iron stores depleted ~ 6months
  - Recommendation: add iron-containing foods
  - Exclusive breast feeding □ iron deficiency

Achoubey/Wikipedia

Iron Deficiency
Inadequate GI uptake

- Malabsorption
  - Any disease affecting duodenum or acid production
  - Loss of acid □ more Fe3+
  - Status post gastrectomy
  - Proton pump inhibitors
- Rarely malnutrition

Iron Deficiency
Loss of iron

- Bleeding
  - Menorrhagia
  - Peptic ulcers
  - Colon cancer
- Adult or post-menopausal female with iron deficiency must have work-up for colon cancer

Iron Deficiency
Other causes

- Pregnancy
  - "Negative iron balance" in pregnancy
  - Expansion in mothers Hgb mass
  - ↑ demand of fetal growth
  - Prenatal vitamins often contain iron and folate

Øyvind Holmstad/Wikipedia

Pregnancy/OCPs $\%\,Sat = \dfrac{Iron}{TIBC}$

- Increase plasma transferrin
- Percent saturation may be low
- Low ferritin often used to diagnose iron deficiency

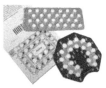

Ceridwen/Wikipedia

Iron Deficiency
Rare causes

- Hookworms
  - Consume blood in intestines
  - Ancylostoma duodenale
  - Necator americanus
- Plummer-Vinson syndrome
  - Rare condition; poorly understood cause
  - Iron deficiency anemia, beefy red tongue, esophageal webs

Pixabay/Public Domain

Iron Deficiency

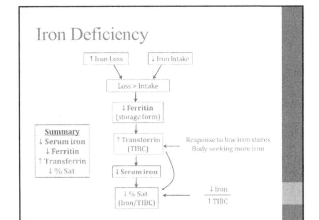

Iron Deficiency Anemia

- Microcytic, hypochromic anemia
  - ↓ RBCs (anemia)
  - Small cells
  - Hypochromic (low hemoglobin)
  - ↓ MCV, MCH, MCHC
- Initially may be normocytic
  - Marrow makes fewer RBCs; maintains Hgb

Red Cell Distribution Width
RDW

- Spectrum of RBC size
- Often wider in iron, B12/Folate deficiency
  - Normal RDW makes iron deficiency unlikely
- Can be normal in mild thalassemia

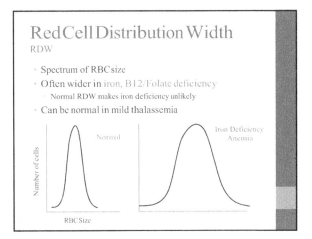

Protoporphyrin

- Heme = Iron + protoporphyrin
- Erythrocyte protoporphyrin level
  - Rarely used blood test
  - Will be elevated in iron deficiency
  - No Fe for protoporphyrin to bind with
- Also elevated in lead poisoning
  - Inhibits addition of iron to protoporphyrin
- Major uses: screening
  - Iron deficiency or lead poisoning

Iron Deficiency Anemia
Treatment

- Iron supplementation
- Usually oral therapy
- Rarely IV iron can be used

Anemia of Chronic Disease

- Anemia in association with inflammation
  - Common in rheumatoid arthritis, lymphoma
  - Many other chronic conditions
- Usually a mild anemia (Hgb > 10g/dL)
- Symptoms from anemia are rare

Anemia of Chronic Disease
Mechanisms

- Triggered by cytokines
- Mild decrease in RBC survival
- Inadequate EPO level/response
  - Lower EPO than expected for degree of anemia
  - Less increase in RBC production by EPO
- Lack of availability of iron
  - Trapped in storage form
  - Key mediator: hepcidin

Hepcidin

- Acute phase protein
  - Produced in liver
  - Has anti-bacterial properties
- Affects iron metabolism
  - Inhibits iron transport
  - Binds to ferroportin in enterocytes, macrophages
- Iron trapped in cells as ferritin
- Contributes to anemia of chronic disease
- Key finding ACD: ↑ferritin

Anemia of Chronic Disease

- Usually normocytic/normochromic
- Microcytic/hypochromic in about 25% cases
  - Low iron availability may lead to small red cells
  - MCV usually mildly decreased (70-80)
- Important to distinguish from iron deficiency
  - Does not respond to iron
- First line therapy: treat underlying disease

Anemia of Chronic Disease
Diagnosis

- Serum iron is low
  - Thought to be protective
  - Bacteria may use iron for growth/metabolism
- Ferritin is usually increased
  - Iron trapped in storage form
  - Ferritin is acute phase reactant
  - Increase may not represent increased storage iron
- Transferrin (TIBC) is usually decreased
  - Transferrin rises when total body iron low
- % saturation usually normal

Iron Studies

	Iron	Ferritin	TIBC	% Sat
Iron Deficiency	↓	↓	↑	↓↓
Anemia Chronic Disease	↓	↑	↓	--
Hemochromatosis	↑	↑	↓	↑↑

Elevated when body storage iron is low

Lead Poisoning

- Exposure to lead:
  - Adults: Inhalation from industrial work (battery factory)
  - Children: Eating lead paint (old house)
- Inhibits heme synthesis via two enzymes in RBCs
  - Delta-aminolevulinic acid (δ-ALA) dehydratase
  - Ferrochelatase
- ↓ heme synthesis ☐ microcytic, hypochromic anemia
- Iron studies: normal or low

Heme Synthesis

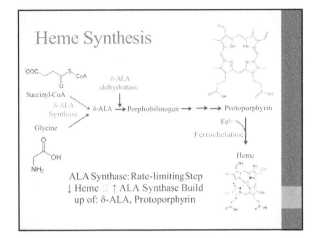

ALA Synthase: Rate-limiting Step
↓ Heme ☐ ↑ ALA Synthase Build
up of: δ-ALA, Protoporphyrin

Lead Poisoning
Diagnosis

- Plasma lead level
- ↑ delta-aminolevulinic acid(δ-ALA)
- ↑ erythrocyte protoporphyrin

Lead Poisoning
Diagnosis

- Blood smear: basophilic stippling
  - Blue granules in cytoplasm of red cells
  - Lead inhibits pyrimidine 5' nucleotidase
  - Normally digests pyrimidines in ribosomes/RNA
  - Leads to accumulation of pyrimidines/RNA in RBCs
- Also seen in thalassemia, other anemias

isis325/Flikr

Lead Poisoning
Symptoms

- Abdominal pain ("lead colic")
- Constipation
- Headache
- "Lead lines"
  - Blue pigment a gum-tooth line
  - Caused by reaction of lead with dental plaque
- Nephropathy
  - Injury to proximal tubules (Fanconi-type syndrome)
  - Glucose, amino acids, and phosphate wasting
- Neuropathy
  - Common symptom: Drop wrist and foot

Lead Poisoning
Symptoms

- Children may have prominent neurologic effects
  - Behavioral issues
  - Developmental delay
  - Failure to reach milestones (i.e. language)
- Many states screen children with lead level testing
  - Usually at 1-2 years of age

Lead Poisoning
Treatment

- Removal of exposure to lead
- Chelation therapy
  - Dimercaprol (2,3-dimercapto-1-propanol)
  - Calcium disodium EDTA (ethylenediaminetetraacetate)
  - DMSA (2,3-dimercaptosuccinic acid; succimer)

Sideroblastic Anemia

- Sideroblasts:
  - Found in normal bone marrow
  - Nucleated red cell precursors
  - Contain granules with non-heme iron
- Sideroblastic anemia
  - Usually microcytic anemia
  - Sideroblasts in peripheral blood

Paulo Henrique Orlandi Mourao

Sideroblastic Anemia

- Failure to make protoporphyrin
- Iron cannot bind ☐ heme
- Iron accumulation in mitochondria

OOC $\overset{O}{\underset{}{}}$ S-CoA

Succinyl-CoA

Glycine

δ-ALA ⟶ ⟶ Protoporphyrin

$Fe^?$ ⟶ Heme

$\overset{O}{\underset{NH_2}{}}$OH

Sideroblastic Anemia

- Usually secondary to a toxin
  - Alcohol (mitochondrial poison)
  - Vitamin B6 deficiency (Isoniazid)
  - Lead poisoning (controversial)

OOC $\overset{O}{\underset{}{}}$ S-CoA

Succinyl-CoA

B6 ⟶ δ-ALA Synthase ⟶ δ-ALA ⟶ ⟶ ⟶ ⟶ Heme

Glycine

$\overset{O}{\underset{NH_2}{}}$OH

Sideroblastic Anemia

- X-linked sideroblastic anemia
  - Rare, inherited deficiency of ALA synthase
  - Most common hereditary sideroblastic anemia
- Often responds to treatment with vitamin B6

OOC $\overset{O}{\underset{}{}}$ S-CoA

Succinyl-CoA

B6 ⟶ δ-ALA Synthase ⟶ δ-ALA ⟶ ⟶ ⟶ Heme

Glycine

$\overset{O}{\underset{NH_2}{}}$OH

Sideroblastic Anemia
Lab Findings

- Microcytic, hypochromic anemia
- Iron studies show iron overload
  - ↑ serum iron
  - ↑ ferritin
  - ↓ TIBC (transferrin)
- Low erythrocyte protoporphyrin levels

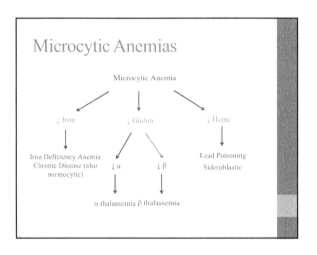

Thalassemias

Jason Ryan, MD, MPH

Anemia Classification

- MCV commonly used to classify anemias

Microcytic MCV<80	Normocytic MCV 80-100	Macrocytic MCV>100
Iron deficiency	Iron deficiency	Folate/B12 deficiency
Anemia Chronic Disease	Anemia Chronic Disease	Orotic Aciduria
Thalassemia	Hemolysis	Liver disease
Lead poisoning	Aplastic anemia	Alcoholism
Sideroblastic Anemia	Kidney disease	Reticulocytosis

Microcytic Anemias

- Usually due to ↓ hemoglobin in red cells
- Usually associated with ↓ MCH and MCHC
- Low hemoglobin ▢ hypochromic RBCs on smear

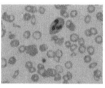

Roberto J. Galindo

Thalassemia

- Decreased or absent production of globin chains
  - Alpha thalassemia: alpha globin
  - Beta thalassemia: beta globin

Globins and Hemoglobin

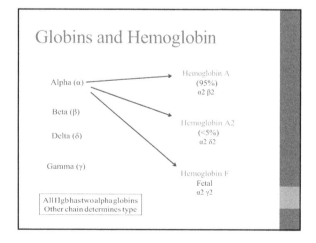

Alpha (α) → Hemoglobin A (95%) α2 β2

Beta (β) → Hemoglobin A2 (<5%) α2 δ2

Delta (δ)

Gamma (γ) → Hemoglobin F Fetal α2 γ2

All Hgb has two alpha globins
Other chain determines type

Globins and Hemoglobin

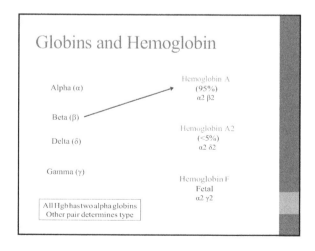

Alpha (α)

Beta (β) → Hemoglobin A (95%) α2 β2

Delta (δ)   Hemoglobin A2 (<5%) α2 δ2

Gamma (γ)   Hemoglobin F Fetal α2 γ2

All Hgb has two alpha globins
Other pair determines type

Globins and Hemoglobin

Alpha (α)

Beta (β)

Delta (δ)

Gamma (γ)

Hemoglobin A
(95%)
α2 β2

Hemoglobin A2
(<5%)
α2 δ2

Hemoglobin F
Fetal
α2 γ2

All Hgb has two alpha globins
Other pair determines type

Hgb Electrophoresis

- Electrical charge applied to sample on gel
- Different hemoglobin □ different distances moved
- Determines HgbA, HgbA2, HgbF, HgbS
- Used to diagnose hemoglobinopathies
  - Thalassemia
  - Sickle cell disease

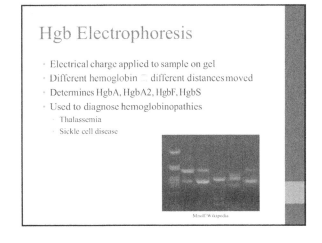

MmdE Wikipedia

Thalassemia

- Spectrum of severity
- Thalassemia minor
  - Often asymptomatic
  - Identified on routine blood testing or blood smear
- Thalassemia major
  - Severe loss of globin production
  - Lifelong transfusions or death

Alpha Thalassemia

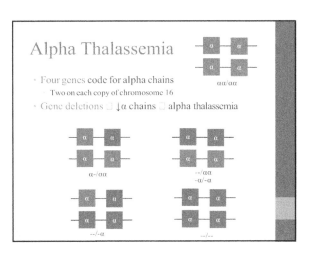

- Four genes code for alpha chains
  - Two on each copy of chromosome 16

  αα/αα
- Gene deletions □ ↓α chains □ alpha thalassemia

α-/αα

--/αα
-α/-α

--/-α

--/--

Alpha Thalassemia Minima

- Normal red cells
- No symptoms
- Carrier state

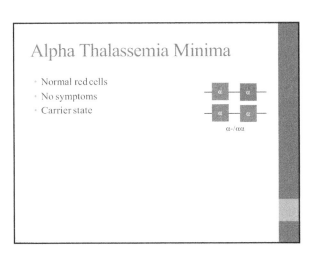

α-/αα

Alpha Thalassemia Minor
Alpha Thalassemia Trait

- No symptoms
- Can have normal red cells
- Sometimes mild anemia
  - ↓ MCV/MCH/MCHC

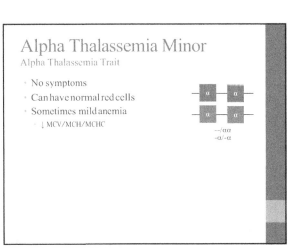

--/αα
-α/-α

Alpha Thalassemia Minor
Alpha Thalassemia Trait

- Common among Asians and Africans
- Alpha minor can be cis (αα/--) or trans (α-/α-)
- Asians more commonly have cis type
- Africans: trans

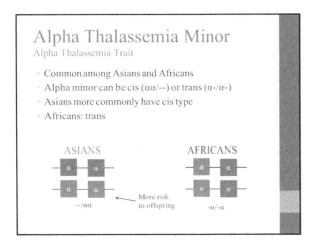

ASIANS
--/αα

More risk to offspring

AFRICANS
-α/-α

HbH Disease

- Very little alpha globin production
- Excess beta globin
- HbH forms: 4 beta chains
  - Easily damaged
  - Affinity for oxygen 10x HbA
  - Useless for oxygen delivery
- HbH forms after birth
  - No β chains in HbF
  - More β produced ☐ HbH

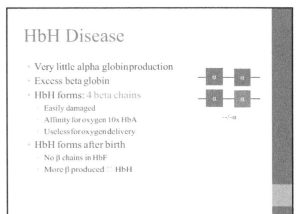

--/-α

HbH Disease

- Hypochromic, microcytic anemia
- Low MCV, MCH, MCHC

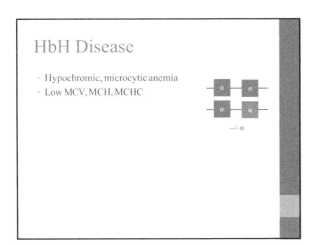

--/-α

HbH Disease

- Abnormal RBC deformability
- Extravascular hemolysis
  - Splenomegaly
  - Indirect hyperbilirubinemia
  - Elevated LDH
- HBH easily oxidized
  - Risk for intravascular hemolysis
  - Occurs with oxidant stressors (infection, drugs)
  - Similar glucose-6-phosphate dehydrogenase deficiency

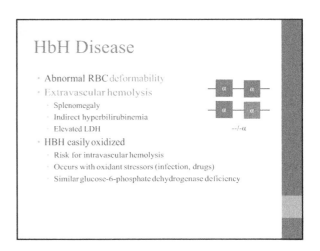

--/-α

HbH Disease

- Diagnosis: DNA testing
- Electrophoresis insensitive
  - Some production A and A2
  - May see HbH depending on amount

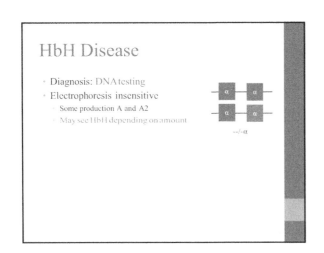

--/-α

HbH Disease

- Treatment:
  - Splenectomy
  - Transfusions
- Long term risk: iron overload

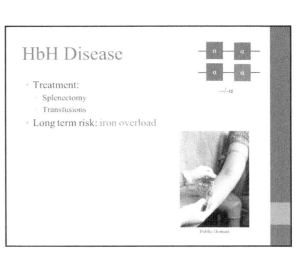

--/-α

Public Domain

Hgb Barts

- No α globin
- Cannot form HbF
- Hgb Barts forms in utero
  - Four gamma globin chains
- Cannot release oxygen to tissues
  - Affinity for oxygen 10x HbA
- Hydrops fetalis
  - Massive total body edema
  - High output heart failure
- Fetal death usually occurs or death hours after birth

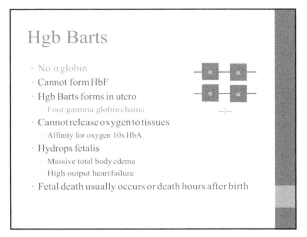

Beta Thalassemia

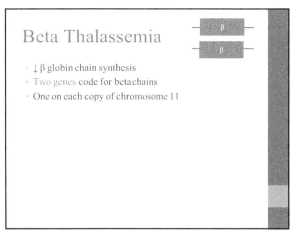

- ↓ β globin chain synthesis
- Two genes code for beta chains
- One on each copy of chromosome 11

Beta Thalassemia

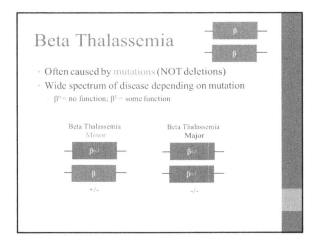

- Often caused by mutations (NOT deletions)
- Wide spectrum of disease depending on mutation
  - β^0 = no function; β^1 = some function

Beta Thalassemia Minor   Beta Thalassemia Major

β_{0x1} β_{0x1}

β β_{0x1}

+/-   -/-

Beta Thalassemia

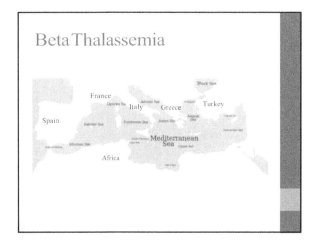

Beta Thalassemia Minor

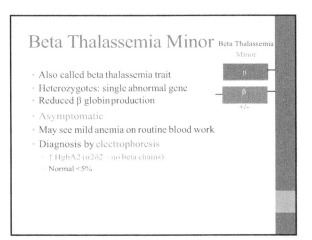

Beta Thalassemia Minor

- Also called beta thalassemia trait
- Heterozygotes: single abnormal gene
- Reduced β globin production
- Asymptomatic
- May see mild anemia on routine blood work
- Diagnosis by electrophoresis
  - ↑ HgbA2 (α2δ2 - no beta chains)
  - Normal <5%

Beta Thalassemia Major

Cooley's Anemia

- No or severely limited β globin production
- Anemia beginning 1st year of life
  - HgbF (α2γ2) production wanes
- Ineffective erythropoiesis
  - Alpha chains form tetramers
  - Precipitate □ RBC damage
  - Failure to produce RBCs
- Splenomegaly
  - Spleen clears any abnormal RBCs in plasma

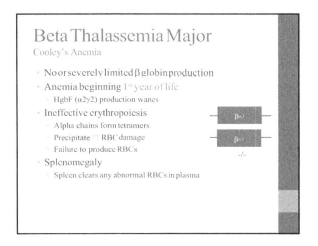

Beta Thalassemia Major
Cooley's Anemia

- Hypochromic, microcytic anemia
- Abnormal red blood cells shapes
- Erythroid hyperplasia
- Extramedullary hematopoiesis

RBC Abnormalities

- Microcytosis (small RBCs)
- Hypochromia (loss of Hgb)
- Anisocytosis
  - Wide variation in sizes of RBCs
  - Increased red cell distribution width (RDW)
- Poikilocytosis (abnormal shapes)
- Basophilic stippling
- Nucleated RBCs
- Target cells

Basophilic Stippling

- Residual RNA in red cells
- Often seen with nucleated RBC
- Seen in thalassemia
- Also lead poisoning

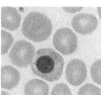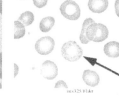

Prasad CSBR   isis325 Flikr

Target Cells

- Target formed in center of RBC
  - Small dark area in center of cell
- Due to ↑ surface area-to-volume ratio
- Extra cell membrane □ target appearance

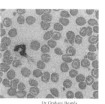

Dr Graham Beards

Target Cells

- Decreased cell volume
  - Thalassemia
  - Can be seen in iron deficiency
- Increased cell membrane
  - Liver disease (↑ cholesterol in membrane)
  - Splenic dysfunction (↓ removal excess membranes)

Erythroid Hyperplasia

- Massive expansion of bone marrow
- ↑↑ EPO without normal response
- Consequence of severe anemia in beta major disease
- Abnormalities of skull and facial bones
  - "Chipmunk facies"
  - Crew cut appearance of skull on x-ray
- Delayed skeletal maturation
- Widening of marrow spaces □ osteoporosis

Extramedullary hematopoiesis

- Hematopoiesis outside of bone marrow
- Consequence of severe anemia in beta major disease
- Liver and spleen produce RBCs
- Hepatosplenomegaly
- Often produces nucleated RBCs

Parvovirus B19

- Infection may cause aplastic crisis
- Beta major patients highly dependent bone marrow

B19

Beta Thalassemia Major
Cooley's Anemia

- Diagnosis: Electrophoresis
- Increased Hgb forms that do not require beta chains
- ↓ or absent HbA (α2β2)
- ↑ HbA2 (α2δ2)
- ↑ HbF (α2γ2)

Beta Thalassemia Major
Cooley's Anemia

- Treatment: Blood transfusions
- Long term risk: iron overload

Public Domain

Beta Thalassemia Intermedia

- Symptomatic beta thalassemia
- Does not require transfusions
- Chronic hemolytic anemia
- Bone marrow expansion
- Hepatosplenomegaly

Malaria

- Alpha and beta thalassemia protective vs. malaria
- ↓ growth in RBCs of plasmodium falciparum

Trophozoite Ring

CDC/Public Domain

Red Cell Distribution Width

RDW

- Spectrum of RBC size
- Wider in iron deficiency
- Can be normal in mild thalassemia
- Normal RDW makes iron deficiency unlikely

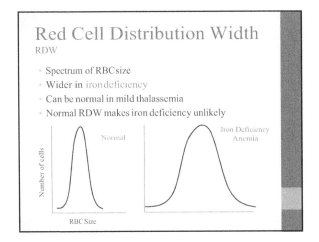

Thalassemia

Key Points

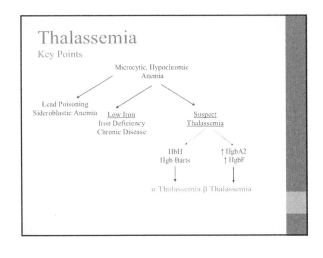

Sickle Cell Anemia

Jason Ryan, MD, MPH

Normocytic Anemias

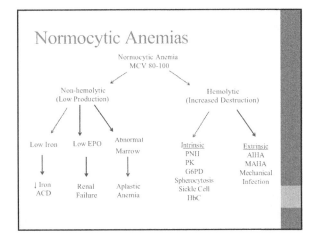

Normocytic Anemia
MCV 80-100

Non-hemolytic (Low Production)
- Low Iron → ↓ Iron ACD
- Low EPO → Renal Failure
- Abnormal Marrow → Aplastic Anemia

Hemolytic (Increased Destruction)
- Intrinsic: PNH, PK, G6PD, Spherocytosis, Sickle Cell, HbC
- Extrinsic: AIHA, MAHA, Mechanical Infection

Sickle Cell Anemia

- Autosomal recessive disorder
- Abnormal β hemoglobin chains
  - Beta chains found in hemoglobin A (α2 β2)
  - Makes up 95% of Hgb

Sickle Cell Anemia

- Root cause is abnormal beta globin gene
- Single base substitution 6th codon of β gene
- Adenine changed to thymine
- Abnormal genes produce HbS

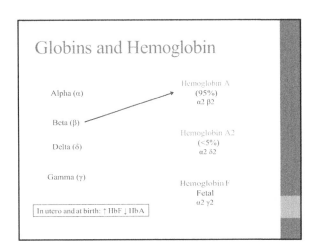

Sickle Cell Trait
βS → HbS (α2S2)
β → HbA (α2β2)

Sickle Cell Disease
βS, βS → HbS (α2S2)

Sickle Cell Anemia

- Substitution of valine for glutamate in beta chains
  - Glutamate: polar (hydrophilic)
  - Valine: non-polar (hydrophobic)
- Alters shape of beta chains

Valine (HbS)

Glutamate (Normal Hgb)

Globins and Hemoglobin

Alpha (α)

Beta (β)

Delta (δ)

Gamma (γ)

Hemoglobin A (95%) α2 β2

Hemoglobin A2 (<5%) α2 δ2

Hemoglobin F Fetal α2 γ2

In utero and at birth: ↑ HbF ↓ HbA

Sickle Cell Anemia

- Deoxygenated HbS is poorly soluble
- Polymerization when O2 low
  - Also in dehydration, acidosis
- Red blood cells form crescents
- Appearance of a sickle
- Causes a ↓ESR

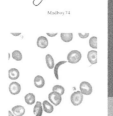

Madboy74

Scooterdma/Flikr

Sickle Cell Anemia

- Two major problems result from sickle cells
- #1: Hemolytic anemia
- #2: Vaso-occlusion of small blood vessels

Sickle Cell Anemia
Hemolysis

- Sickling is reversible
- Cells continuously sickle/de-sickle in circulation
- Over time this leads to RBC membrane damage
- Results in extravascular hemolysis
  - Anemia
  - Jaundice
  - Elevated unconjugated bilirubin
  - Pigment gallstones
- Some intravascular hemolysis may also occur

Sickle Cell Anemia
Erythroid Hyperplasia

- ↑↑ EPO
- Massive expansion of bone marrow
- Consequence of severe anemia:
  - Also seen in beta thalassemia major
- Abnormalities of skull and facial bones
  - "Chipmunk facies"
  - Crew cut appearance of skull on x-ray
- Delayed skeletal maturation
- Widening of marrow spaces ☐ osteoporosis

Sickle Cell Anemia
Parvovirus B19

- Infection may cause aplastic crisis
- Crisis also seen in spherocytosis, thalassemia

B19

Sickle Cell Anemia
Vaso-occlusion

- Sickle cells may occlude microvasculature
- May affect any organ
- Classic clinical manifestation:
  - Swollen hands ("dactylitis")
  - Acute pain crises
  - Spleen failure ☐ infections
  - Acute chest syndrome
  - Renal dysfunction

Sickle Cell Anemia
Dactylitis

- Pain/swelling in hands or feet
- Fingers may look like "sausage" digits
- Common initial symptom among children

Sickle Cell Anemia
Avascular Necrosis

- Bone collapse
- Most commonly femoral head
- Also associated with long term steroid use

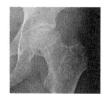

Imarchn/Wikipedia

Sickle Cell Anemia
Pain Crises

- Episodes of acute pain ("sickle cell crisis")
  - Sudden onset of pain
- Most common type of vaso-occlusive event
- May affect any part of body
  - Abdomen, bones, joints, soft tissue, fingers, toes
  - Swollen hands and/or feet especially in children
- Treatment: Hydration and pain medications

Sickle Cell Anemia
Splenic Failure

- Repeated splenic infarctions □ functional asplenia
  - Early in disease: splenomegaly (macrophage hyperplasia)
  - Late in disease: Fibrosis and atrophy
- Howell-Jolly bodies will appear in peripheral blood

Paulo Henrique Orlandi Mourao /Mikael Häggström

Sickle Cell Anemia
Splenic Failure

- Increased risk of infections by encapsulated bacteria
- Strep pneumoniae and H influenza
  - Bacteremia/sepsis from S. Pneumoniae
  - Patients must be vaccinated
- Osteomyelitis from Salmonella species
  - Infection of infarcted bones
  - Most common cause SCA is Salmonella (usually S. Aureus)

Sickle Cell Anemia
Splenic Sequestration Crisis

- Vaso-occlusion in spleen □ pooling of red cells
- Marked fall in hemoglobin level
- Rapidly enlarging spleen
- Risk of hypovolemic shock especially in children
  - Occurs in spleens yet to develop fibrosis
  - May occur before sickle cell disease is diagnosed

Sickle Cell Anemia
Chest Syndrome

- Leading cause of death in adults with SCD
- Vaso-occlusion of pulmonary microvasculature
- Often triggered by infection (pneumonia)
  - Increased sickling in lungs
  - Once begun ⬜ inflammation/acidosis ⬜ more sickling

Sickle Cell Anemia
Chest Syndrome

- Chest pain and shortness of breath
- Infiltrate on chest x-ray
- Looks like pneumonia
- Treatment:
  - Fluids and pain medication (similar to pain crisis)
  - Antibiotics, oxygen, bronchodilators
  - Transfusions as needed

Sickle Cell Anemia
Renal Dysfunction

- Occlusion of vasa recta in renal medulla
  - Medulla has low oxygen and high osmolality
  - Promotes sickling
- May impair concentrating ability
  - Cannot raise urine osmolality even with H_2O deprivation
  - Causes nocturia and polyuria

The Nephron

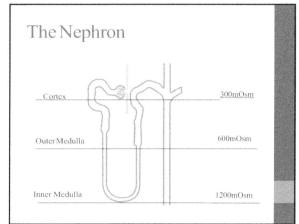

Cortex	300mOsm
Outer Medulla	600mOsm
Inner Medulla	1200mOsm

Sickle Cell Anemia
Renal Dysfunction

- Papillary necrosis
  - Sloughing of renal papilla due to renal vaso-occlusion
  - Usually painless
  - Gross hematuria and proteinuria

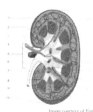

Image courtesy of Piotr Michał Jaworski

Sickle Cell Anemia
Treatment

- Immunizations
- Hydroxyurea
  - Raises amount of HbF
  - Mechanism unclear
- Transfusions
  - Iron overload may develop
- Bone marrow transplant is curative
- Median survival 42-48 years

Sickle Cell Trait

- One mutated beta globin gene
- Usually no sickling
  - Normal beta gene more effective ⊥ >50% beta globins
  - Need >50% HbS for sickling
- One exception: Renal medulla
  - May see loss of concentrating ability
  - ↑ risk of renal medullary carcinoma (> than sickle disease)

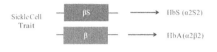

Sickle Cell Diagnosis
Disease or Trait

- Electrophoresis
  - Will show presence of HbS
  - Different amounts disease versus trait
- Sickling Test
  - Sodium metabisulphite reduces the oxygen tension
  - HbS becomes insoluble
  - Forms a turbid suspension ⊔ easily visualized
  - Other hemoglobin types remain in solution
  - Positive if any amount HbS present (disease or trait)

Electrophoresis

	Normal	Sickle Cell Disease	Sickle Cell Trait
HbA	97%	--	55%
HbA2	2%	2%	2%
HbF	1%	2-15%	1%
HbS	--	~90%	40%

Malaria

- Sickle trait protective against p. falciparum
  - Cells sickle when infected ... ↑ clearance
  - Does not protect against infection
  - When infection does occur it is milder
  - Patients still need malaria prophylaxis
- African Americans: 8 to 10% have sickle cell trait
- Sub-Saharan Africa: ~30%

Sickle Cell/Beta Thalassemia

- One beta gene: sickle cell
- One beta gene: beta thalassemia
- Clinical manifestations similar to sickle cell
  - Vary depending on beta thalassemia gene function
  - β⁰: Similar to sickle cell disease
  - β⁺: Less severe

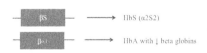

Hemoglobin C

- Rare mutation of beta gene (different from SCA)
- Glutamic acid replaced by lysine (not valine)
- Heterozygotes: Mild anemia (extravascular hemolysis)

Lysine

Glutamate

Hemoglobin C

- Presence of HbC crystals on smear
- Induces red cell dehydration: ↑ MCHC

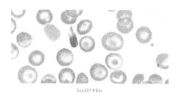

Isto325/Flikr

Hemoglobin SC

- One HbS gene plus one HbC gene
- More common than homozygous HbC disease
- At risk for same complications as sickle cell disease
- Lower frequency of complications

Other Anemias

Jason Ryan, MD, MPH

Anemias

- Microcytic
- Normocytic, hemolytic
- Normocytic, non-hemolytic
- Macrocytic

Normocytic Anemias

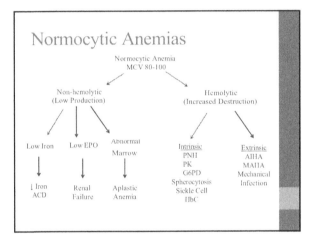

Normocytic Anemia
MCV 80-100

Non-hemolytic (Low Production)

Hemolytic (Increased Destruction)

Low Iron → ↓ Iron ACD
Low EPO → Renal Failure
Abnormal Marrow → Aplastic Anemia

Intrinsic
PNH
PK
G6PD
Spherocytosis
Sickle Cell
HbC

Extrinsic
AIHA
MAHA
Mechanical
Infection

EPO
Erythropoietin

- Synthesized in the kidney
  - Interstitial cells peritubular capillary
  - Found in cortex of the kidney
- Released in response to hypoxia
- Decreased production in renal failure
- Results in a normocytic anemia

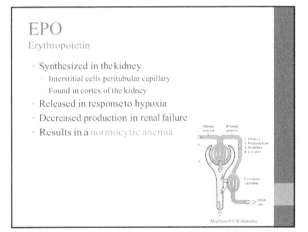

Madhero88/Wikipedia

Kidney Anatomy

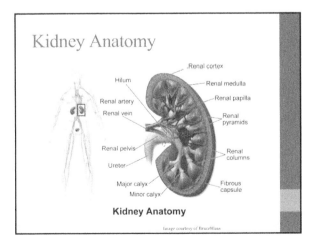

- Renal cortex
- Hilum
- Renal medulla
- Renal papilla
- Renal artery
- Renal vein
- Renal pyramids
- Renal pelvis
- Renal columns
- Ureter
- Major calyx
- Minor calyx
- Fibrous capsule

Kidney Anatomy

Image courtesy of BruceBlaus

EPO Injections

- Darbepoetin alfa (Aranesp)
- Epoetin alfa (Epogen)
- Used to treat anemia of chronic kidney disease
- FDA Black Box warning
- Generally reserved for patients with severe anemia

Aplastic Anemia

- Loss of hematopoietic precursors in bone marrow
- Results in pancytopenia
  - ↓ WBC, ↓ Platelets, ↓ RBC

Vocabulary

- "Aplasia": Defective or absent development
- Bone marrow failure
  - Bone marrow cannot produce cells
  - Results in pancytopenia
  - Many causes: fibrosis, tumors
  - "Myelophthisis:" displacement of bone-marrow tissue
- Aplastic anemia:
  - Specific type of bone marrow failure
  - Defective stem cells ⇒ acellular/hypocellular bone marrow

Aplastic Anemia
Hallmarks

- Pancytopenia
- Acellular or hypocellular bone marrow
  - Bone marrow biopsy for diagnosis
  - Absence of cells/replacement with fat

Chalm Drosera

Aplastic Anemia
Symptoms

- Pancytopenia (normal cells but not enough)
- Anemia
  - Fatigue, pallor
- Thrombocytopenia
  - Bleeding
- Leukopenia
  - Infections

Aplastic Anemia
Causes

- Most commonly idiopathic
- Radiation
- Drugs
- Viruses
- Inherited (Fanconi anemia)

Aplastic Anemia
Idiopathic

- Unknown trigger
- Strong evidence for immune mediated mechanism
- T-cell mediated destruction of stem cells

Aplastic Anemia
Idiopathic

- Can be treated with immunosuppression
- Antithymocyte globulin
    - Animal-derived antibodies against human T cells
    - Usually from rabbits or horses
    - Also can be used in kidney transplant patients
- Cyclosporine

Aplastic Anemia
Radiation

- Well-described cause of aplastic anemia
- Radiation □ damage to stem cells □ aplastic anemia

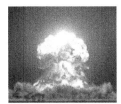

Public Domain

Aplastic Anemia
Chemicals

- Benzene: well-described cause of aplastic anemia
- Rubber factories, shoe repair shops
- Often with poor ventilation

Aplastic Anemia
Drugs

- Most cancer therapies
    - Anticipated effect
- Chloramphenicol
    - Rarely used antibiotic (bacterial protein synthesis inhibitor)
- Phenylbutazone
    - Old NSAID
    - Pulled from market due to cases of aplastic anemia
- Methimazole, Propylthiouracil (PTU)
    - Aplastic anemia cases reported (monitor WBCs)

Aplastic Anemia
Viruses

- Parvovirus B19
    - Infects proerythroblasts
    - Usually causes ↓ RBCs ("red cell aplasia")
    - Pancytopenia can occur
    - ↑ risk: immunocompromised

Aplastic Anemia
Viruses

- Acute Viral Hepatitis
    - Can cause aplastic anemia
    - Reported after infection with HAV, HBV, HCV, HDV, and HEV
    - Often affects boys and young adult males
    - Aplasia develops weeks to months after acute hepatitis
- Others: HIV, EBV, CMV
- All probably NOT caused directly by virus
- Evidence suggests T-cell activation

Fanconi Anemia

- Inherited aplastic anemia
- Autosomal recessive or X-linked
- Usually presents in children <16 years old
- More than half of patients have physical deformities
  - Short stature
  - Cafe-au-lait spots
  - Malformed thumbs
  - Heart, renal, eye abnormalities described

Fanconi Anemia

- More than 13 genetic abnormalities identified
- Many involve DNA repair enzymes
  - Hypersensitivity to DNA damage
  - Especially vulnerable to abnormal DNA strand cross-links
- Increased risk of malignancies
  - Myelodysplastic syndrome (MDS)
  - Acute myeloid leukemia (AML)
  - Squamous cell carcinoma of head, neck or vulva

Aplastic Anemia
Treatment

- Stop offending agent
- Transfusions (red cells, platelets)
- Bone marrow stimulation
  - EPO, GM-CSF, G-CSF
- Immunosuppression
  - Antithymocyte globulin
  - Cyclosporine
- Bone marrow transplant

Pure Red Cell Aplasia

- Absence of erythroid precursors in bone marrow
- Marked reduction in reticulocytes
- Normal granulocytes, platelets
- Usually idiopathic
- Associated with some drugs, viral infections
- Key association: Thymoma
  - Present in 5 percent of PRCA cases

Macrocytic Anemias

- MCV > 100
- Abnormal DNA synthesis
  - "Megaloblastic anemias"
- Other
  - Liver disease, alcohol, reticulocytosis

Megaloblastic anemias

- Red blood cell precursors grow but cannot divide
  - Contrast with microcytic anemias: divide too much
- Results from abnormal DNA synthesis
  - Cells cannot efficiently make DNA for cellular division

Megaloblastic Anemias

- Anemia (↓Hct)
- Large RBCs (↑MCV)
- Hypersegmented neutrophils
  - WBCs also cannot divide effectively due to ↓DNA synthesis
  - Result: hypersegmentation of nucleus (>5 lobes)

Wikipedia/Public Domain

Megaloblastic Anemias

- Causes of defective DNA production
  - Folate deficiency
  - B12
  - Orotic aciduria
  - Drugs (MTX, 5-FU, hydroxyurea)
  - Zidovudine (HIV NRTIs)

Wikipedia/Public Domain

Macrocytic Anemias
Non-megaloblastic

- Macrocytosis without impaired DNA synthesis
- Liver disease
  - Exact mechanism not known
  - Increased lipids seen in red cell membranes
- Alcoholism
  - Common cause of macrocytosis
  - Acetaldehyde may induce membrane changes in RBCs

```
    H  H                   H
    |  |      O            |      O
H—C—C—O  H     ———>   H—C—C
    |  |                   |      H
    H  H   Alcohol         H
Ethanol  Dehydrogenase  Acetaldehyde
```

Reticulocytosis

- Reticulocytes have MCV of 103 to 126fl
- Normal RBCs: 80 to 96 fL
- In theory may cause macrocytosis
  - But only about 20% bigger than normal cells
  - Need LOTS of reticulocytes to raise average MCV >100
  - Usually raise average MCV but should not reach >100

Blood Groups

Jason Ryan, MD, MPH

Blood Groups

- Antibodies form to RBC antigens
- "Blood group" defined by RBC antigens
- Important for safely administering blood transfusions
- Must match transfusion to "blood type"
- Two major blood groupings:
  - ABO system
  - Rh system

ABO System

- A and B antigens can be found on RBCs
- Patients who lack A or B generate antibodies
  - Appear in blood by 4-6 months
  - Exposure to bacterial antigens with similar structure
  - Occurs as the gut becomes colonized
- Antibodies: IgM
- Do not cross placenta
- Key point: A and B antibodies are naturally occurring

ABO System

	Group A	Group B	Group AB	Group O
Red blood cell type	A	B	AB	O
Antibodies in Plasma	Anti-B	Anti-A	None	Anti-A and Anti-B
Antigens in Red Blood Cell	A antigen	B antigen	A and B antigens	None

InvictaHOG/Wikipedia/Public Domain

ABO System

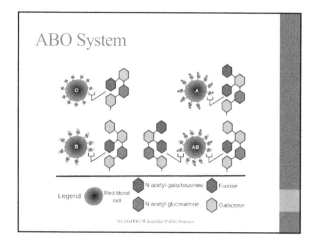

Legend: Red blood cell, N-acetyl-galactosamine, N-acetyl-glucosamine, Fucose, Galactose

InvictaHOG/Wikipedia/Public Domain

Rh System

- Most important blood group system after ABO
- More than 50 antigens are part of Rh system
  - Names for letters following AB: C, D, E
- All are transmembrane proteins

Rh System

- Presence/absence of D antigen is critical
  - D antigen highly immunogenic
  - "Rh positive:" has the D antigen (of the Rh system)
  - "Rh negative:" lacks the D antigen (of the Rh system)
- Other Rh antigens not routinely tested: C, c, E, e

Rh System

- Rh positivity is common
  - Caucasians: 83%
  - Some Asian populations: 98%
- Rh negative may develop anti-D antibodies
- Only happens if exposed to D⁺ RBC
  - Transfusion
  - Pregnancy (Mom D⁻ with baby D⁺)
- Anti-D antibodies: IgG
- May cross placenta

Newborn Hemolytic Disease

- Classically caused by anti-D (anti-Rh) antibodies
- Can only occur in D⁻ mother with D⁺ baby
- D⁻ mother capable of developing anti-D antibodies
- If father is D⁺: baby may also be D⁺

Newborn Hemolytic Disease

- First pregnancy: Mother exposed D⁺ RBCs at delivery
- 2nd pregnancy: Anti-D IgG in mother → fetus
- If 2nd baby also D⁺ hemolysis will occur in utero

Newborn Hemolytic Disease

- Mild cases present as hemolytic anemia
- Severe cases: Hydrops fetalis
- Massive edema: Pleural/pericardial effusion, ascites
- Mechanisms:
  - High-output congestive heart failure
  - ↑ RBC production by spleen/liver → obstruction
  - Results in portal hypertension
- Seen in other severe anemias of newborns
  - Hgb Barts (lack of alpha globins)

Maternal Antibody Screening
Indirect Coombs Test

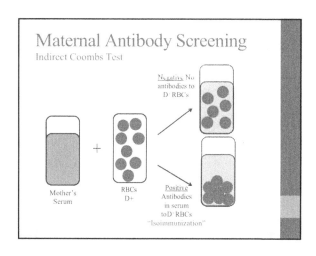

Negative No antibodies to D⁻ RBCs

Mother's Serum + RBCs D+

Positive Antibodies in serum to D⁻ RBCs "Isoimmunization"

Newborn Hemolytic Disease
Prevention

- Anti-D immune globulin ("RhoGAM")
- IgG antibodies to D antigen
- Rapid macrophage clearance of D⁺ RBCs
- Given in 3rd trimester to D⁻ women
- Blocks/prevents isoimmunization

Other Antigens

- Only ABO and Rh routinely tested
- Many other antigens on RBCs
- Only tested when patient has abnormal screening test
- Antibodies from pregnancy or transfusion

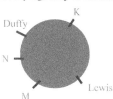

Transfusion Medicine
Common Tests

- Blood type (usually done with another test)
- Type and screen
  - Antibody screening test
  - Further testing if positive
- Type and crossmatch ("type and cross")
  - Matching of donor blood to patient

Blood Type Testing

- Patient RBCs plus antibodies
  - Anti-A; Anti-B; Anti-D
- Agglutination indicates presence of antigen

Blood Type Testing

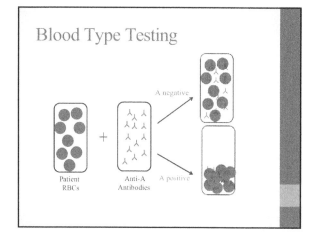

Type and Screen

- Recipient serum plus standard RBCs
- Screen for patient antibodies to rare antigens
- Will only have antibodies if prior exposure
- Reagent RBCs contain many RBC antigens
  - No agglutination: Patient lacks antibodies
  - Agglutination: Antibodies to less common antigens present

Type and Screen

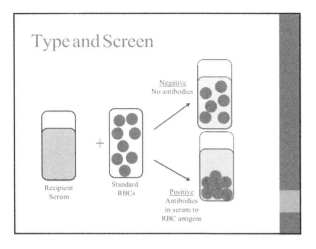

Negative
No antibodies

Recipient Serum

Standard RBCs

Positive
Antibodies
in serum to
RBC antigens

Abnormal Screen

- Determine which antibody is present
- Test patient's serum against large panel of antigens
- Subsequent transfusions: Test donor blood for antigen
- Challenging in patients with long transfusion history
  - Sickle cell anemia
  - Beta thalassemia major
- Key point: Don't transfuse unless necessary

Type and Cross

- Patient serum with potential donor RBC's
- Final test of product to be transfused

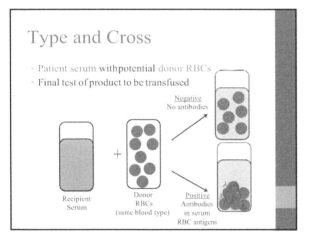

Negative
No antibodies

Recipient Serum

Donor RBCs
(same blood type)

Positive
Antibodies
in serum
RBC antigens

Blood Products

- Packed RBCs
  - RBCs with plasma removed
  - Usually administered instead of "whole blood"
  - Minimizes volume given to patient
- Platelets
  - Express ABO and HLA class I antigens
  - Do not express Rh or HLA class II
  - Reactions from mismatch less common that with RBCs

Blood Products

- Fresh Frozen Plasma (FFP)
  - Plasma after removal of RBC, WBC, and platelets
  - Frozen for storage
  - Once thawed, must be used within 24hrs
  - Clotting factors degrade
  - Corrects deficiencies of any clotting factor
  - PT/PTT will normalize after infusion
- Cryoprecipitate
  - Precipitate that forms when FFP is thawed
  - Contains lots of fibrinogen
  - Massive bleeding or rare ↓ fibrinogen disorders

Transfusion Reactions

- Acute hemolytic reaction
- Anaphylaxis
- Febrile reaction
- TRALI
- Many, many other potential reactions
  - Heart failure
  - Sepsis

AHTR
Acute hemolytic transfusion reaction

- Feared complication of blood transfusion
- Pre-formed antibodies ⊐ donor RBCs
  - Type II hypersensitivity reaction
  - Usually from transfusion of incorrect blood product

AHTR
Acute hemolytic transfusion reaction

- Life-threatening reaction
- Acute hemolysis of transfused RBCs
  - Intravascular (complement; anti-AB are IgM)
  - Extravascular (spleen)
- Can lead to DIC
- Fever, chills, flank pain, oozing from intravenous sites
- Jaundice, elevated bilirubin ⊐ dark urine
- Direct antiglobulin test (Coombs) will be positive

AHTR
Acute hemolytic transfusion reaction

- Usual cause: system or clerical error
- Transfusion of wrong blood product
- Numerous safety measures used to prevent:
  - Blood type, antibody screen, cross match
  - Careful patient identification

Anaphylaxis

- Allergic reaction (type I hypersensitivity)
- Hives, angioedema, wheezing, hypotension
- May occur in IgA-deficient individuals
  - Produce anti-IgA antibodies
  - React with IgA in transfused product
- Also occurs to plasma proteins in transfused product
- Treatment:
  - Stop transfusion
  - Epinephrine, anti-histamines

FNHTR
Febrile non-hemolytic transfusion reaction

- Fever, chills
- No other systemic symptoms
- Caused by cytokines in blood products
  - Especially IL-1
  - Generated by WBCs during storage
  - Accumulate in stored blood components
- Some blood products undergo "leukoreduction"

TRALI
Transfusion-related acute lung injury

- Sudden onset hypoxemia during transfusion
- Inflammatory reaction: Fever, chills are common
- Infiltrates on chest x-ray
- Results from neutrophil activation by blood products
  - Some patients predisposed with PMNs in lungs
  - PMNs release cytokines, reactive oxygen species, enzymes
  - Damage the pulmonary capillary endothelium
  - Exudative fluid loss ⊐ pulmonary edema

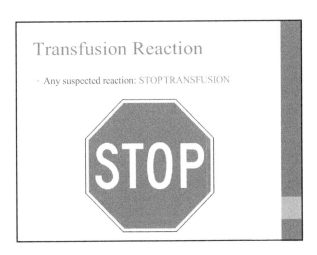

Acute Leukemias

Jason Ryan, MD, MPH

Leukemia

- Malignant proliferation of white blood cells
- Cells appear in blood (contrast with lymphoma)
- Increased WBC

Leukemias
Classification

- Myeloid versus lymphoid
- Acute versus chronic
- Acute
  - Rapid onset of symptoms
  - Involves blasts in bone marrow
- Chronic
  - Slower onset of symptoms (or no symptoms)
  - Malignant cells are not blasts (more mature)

Hematopoiesis

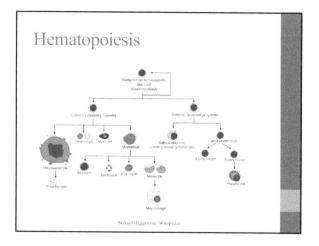

Mikael Häggström, Wikipedia

Myeloid Disorders

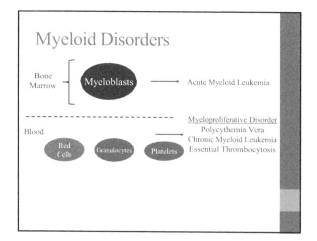

Lymphoid Disorders

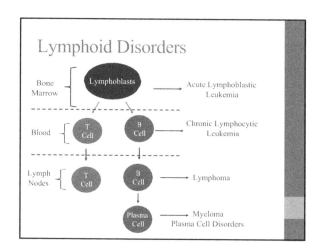

90

ALL
Acute Lymphoblastic Leukemia

- Disease of children
  - Peak incidence ~ 4 years old
- Fever
- Bone pain (marrow expansion)
- Lymphadenopathy, splenomegaly, hepatomegaly
  - Infiltration by malignant cells
- Headache, vomiting
  - Meningeal spread
- May cause bone marrow depression
  - Anemia, thrombocytopenia, neutropenia

ALL
Acute Lymphoblastic Leukemia

- Peripheral blood: lymphoblasts
  - Can appear similar to myeloblasts
  - Special testing distinguish from myeloblasts

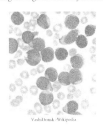

VashiDonsk / Wikipedia

Lymphocyte Development

Stem Cell

CD10

CD19 CD20

TdT+ → B
CD21

CD5 CD8
T CD7
CD2 CD3

CD5 CD7
TdT+
CD2 CD3

CD5 CD4
T CD7
CD2 CD3

Lymphocyte Antigens

Primarily T-Cell Associated	Primarily B-cell Associated
CD1	CD10
CD2	CD19
CD3	CD20
CD4	CD21
CD5	CD22
CD7	CD23
CD8	

ALL
Acute Lymphoblastic Leukemia

- Usually pre-B cell malignancy (~70 to 80% cases)
  - CD10
  - "Common acute lymphoblastic leukemia antigen" or "CALLA"
  - Also CD19+, sometimes CD20+
- Terminal dexoytransferase (TdT)
  - DNA polymerase (found in nucleus)
  - Found only in pre-B and pre-T blasts
  - NOT seen in myeloblasts

ALL
Acute Lymphoblastic Leukemia

- Treated with chemotherapy
  - Cure rates >80% in many studies
- "Sanctuary sites"
  - Poor penetration by chemotherapy drugs
  - Relapse may occur in these locations
- Testes
- Central nervous system
- Special treatments (radiation/chemo) used
- Sterility may occur in boys

ALL
Acute Lymphoblastic Leukemia

- Many different translocations reported in B-ALL
- Philadelphia chromosome t(9;22)
  - 20 to 30% ALL in adults
  - 2 to 3 % ALL in children
  - Associated with a poor prognosis
- t(12;21)
  - Fusion product of two genes: TEL-AML1
  - TEL-AML1 impairs differentiation of blasts
  - Good prognosis
  - Most common rearrangement in children

ALL
Acute Lymphoblastic Leukemia

- Down Syndrome
  - Risk of ALL ↑↑ 10-20x
  - 1-3% ALL cases have Down

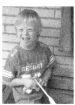

Vanellus Foto/Wikipedia

T-C ell ALL
T-cell acute Lymphoblastic Leukemia

- Less common form of ALL
- Common in adolescent males (teens to 20s)
- Presents as a mass
  - Lymphadenopathy
  - Mediastinal mass
  - Anterior with pleural effusions
- Tumor compression may occur
  - Superior vena cava syndrome
  - Tracheal obstruction

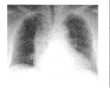

G. Ferretti

T-C ell ALL
T-cell acute Lymphoblastic Leukemia

- Pathology: Blasts
- Different markers from B-cell ALL
  - Usually CD7+
  - Can see CD2, CD3, CD5, CD4, CD8
  - Not CD10+

AML
Acute Myelogenous Leukemia

- Malignancy of myeloblasts
- Common in adult males
  - Median age at diagnosis: 65
  - Male:female ratio: 5:3
- Symptoms from bone marrow suppression
  - Myeloblasts accumulate in marrow, suppress cell growth
  - Anemia: Fatigue, weakness, pallor
  - Thrombocytopenia: Bleeding (especially gums)
  - Neutropenia: Infections
- Enlarged nodes, spleen, liver less common than ALL

AML
Acute Myelogenous Leukemia

- Peripheral blood smear
  - Anemia, thrombocytopenia, blasts
- Myeloblasts
  - Myeloperoxidase (MPO) positive
  - Auer rods

Paulo Henrique Orlandi Mourao Wikipedia

Auer Rods

- Pathognomonic AML
- Accumulation of MPO
- Can cause DIC

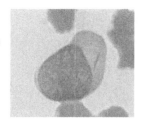

Paulo Henrique Orlandi Mourao Wikipedia

AML
Acute Myelogenous Leukemia

- Classified into numerous subtypes (WHO system)
- Classified by morphology, surface markers, genetics
- Key subtype: APML

APML
Acute Promyelocytic Leukemia

- Defined by translocation t(15;17)
  - Creates a fusion gene: PML-RARA
  - Promyelocytic leukemia gene (chromosome 15)
  - Retinoic acid receptor alpha (chromosome 17)

APML
Acute Promyelocytic Leukemia

- #1: Abnormal retinoic acid receptor (RAR)
  - Prevents normal maturation of promyelocytes
  - Treatment: all trans retinoic acid (form of vitamin A)
  - Abnormal cells will mature

APML
Acute Promyelocytic Leukemia

- #2: Disseminated intravascular coagulation
  - Promyelocytes contains lots of MPO (Auer rods common)
  - Release → DIC (common initial presentation)

Myelodysplasia
Myelodysplastic Syndromes (MDS)

- Abnormal myeloid progenitor cells
- Leads to ineffective hematopoiesis
  - Anemia, thrombocytopenia, neutropenia
- Diagnosis: Bone marrow biopsy
  - Dysplasia (abnormal) cells
  - Blasts <20% cells
- Can progress to AML (>20% blasts)

Vashi Donsk / Wikipedia

| MDS <20% cells blasts | ←———————→ | AML >20% cells blasts |

Myelodysplasia
Myelodysplastic Syndrome (MDS)

- Associated with environmental factors
  - Prior radiation
  - Chemotherapy
  - Usually years after exposure

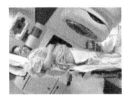

Dina Waktukhih/Wikipedia

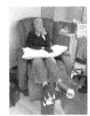

Jenny Mealing/Wikipedia

Chronic Leukemias

Jason Ryan, MD, MPH

Leukemia

- Malignant proliferation of white blood cells
- Cells appear in blood (contrast with lymphoma)
- Increased WBC

Leukemias
Classification

- Myeloid versus lymphoid
- Acute versus chronic
- Acute
  - Rapid onset of symptoms
  - Involves blasts in bone marrow
- Chronic
  - Slower onset of symptoms (or no symptoms)
  - Malignant cells are not blasts (more mature)

Myeloid Disorders

Bone Marrow — Myeloid Progenitor → Myeloblasts → Acute Myeloid Leukemia

Blood — Red Cells, Granulocytes, Platelets

Myeloproliferative Disorder
Polycythemia Vera
Chronic Myeloid Leukemia
Essential Thrombocytosis

CML
Chronic Myelogenous Leukemia

- Malignant disorder of myeloid progenitor cells
- Dysregulated production of granulocytes
  - Neutrophils, basophils, eosinophils
- Classified as a myeloproliferative disorder

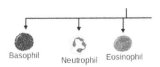

Basophil   Neutrophil   Eosinophil

CML
Chronic Myelogenous Leukemia

- Peripheral blood (chronic phase):
  - Leukocytosis (median WBC 100,000/microL.)
  - ↑ neutrophils
  - ↑ myeloblasts, promyelocytes, myelocytes, bands
  - ↑ basophils (rare finding!)
  - ↑ eosinophils
- Mild anemia; normal or increased platelets

Paulo Henrique Orlandi Mourao/Wikipedia

CML
Chronic Myelogenous Leukemia

- Chronic phase (usually years)
  - Can be asymptomatic (↑WBC on blood testing)
  - Fatigue, malaise, weight loss, splenomegaly
  - Few blasts (usually <2%)
- Accelerated phase (usually months)
  - Treatment failure (rising WBC)
- Blast crisis
  - Acute leukemia (>20% blasts in periphery or marrow)
  - Usually myeloblasts (AML)
  - Less commonly lymphoblasts (ALL)

Left Shift
Leukemoid Reaction

- Normal response to infection
- More bands and neutrophils
- Must be distinguished from CML

	Normal	Infection
WBC	10,000/µL	17,000 /µL
Neutrophils	55%	80%
Bands	5%	12%

LAP
Leukocyte Alkaline Phosphatase

- Enzyme found in normal neutrophils
- Absent in neutrophils of CML
- Enzyme level assessed with LAP score
  - Low = CML
  - High = Leukemoid reaction
- Largely replaced by testing for Ph chromosome

Philadelphia Chromosome

- Genetic hallmark of CML
- 9;22 translocation
- BCR-ABL fusion gene
- Synthesis tyrosine kinase protein
- Long cell life ☐ accumulation

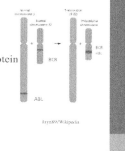

Aryn89/Wikipedia

Tyrosine Kinase Inhibitors
Imatinib, Dasatinib, Nilotinib

- Used for treatment in CML (chronic phase)
- Long term control of disease (not curative)
- Bone marrow transplant often used after failure

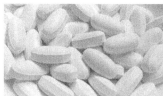

ProjectManhattan/Wikipedia

CLL
Chronic Lymphocytic Leukemia

- Disorder of naïve lymphocytes
  - Not blasts
  - Newly produced by bone marrow
- Characteristic immunophenotype
  - CD5+ B cells
  - "Co-express CD20 and CD5"

SLL
Small lymphocytic lymphoma

- Same malignant cells as CLL
- Differentiated by degree of lymphocytosis (↑WBC)
- CLL: Increased WBC
- SLL: normal or mild lymphocytosis
- SLL definition: lymphocyte count of <5000
- CLL definition: lymphocyte count of >5000

CLL
Chronic Lymphocytic Leukemia

- Median age 60
- Patients often asymptomatic
  - Routine CBC: Increased lymphocytes
  - 5-10% of patients have B symptoms (fevers, sweats)
- Signs
  - Lymphadenopathy, splenomegaly, hepatomegaly
- Many patients observed without treatment

CLL
Chronic Lymphocytic Leukemia

- Smudge cells
  - Peripheral lymphocytes are fragile
  - Disrupted during preparation of blood smear

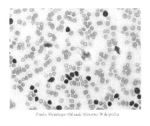

Paulo Henrique Orlandi Mourao/Wikipedia

CLL
Chronic Lymphocytic Leukemia

- B-cell disruption
- Hypogammaglobulinemia
  - Usually ↓ IgG, IgA, IgM
  - Increased susceptibility to bacterial infections
- Autoantibodies
  - Not produced by malignant cells
  - Produced by non-neoplastic cells (self-reactive)
  - Autoimmune hemolytic anemia

CLL
Chronic Lymphocytic Leukemia

- May transform into diffuse large B cell lymphoma
- Classic presentation
  - Patient with known CLL
  - Rapid growth of single lymph node
  - Biopsy: diffuse large B cell lymphoma

Hairy Cell Leukemia

- Rare chronic B-cell malignancy
  - Express CD19, CD20, CD22
  - CD103: sensitive marker
- Peripheral smear: hairy cells
  - Lymphocytes
  - Hair-like cytoplasm projections

Paulo Henrique Orlandi Mourao/Wikipedia

Hairy Cell Leukemia
Unique Features

- Massive splenomegaly
  - Red pulp engorged
  - Atrophy or obliteration of white pulp
- "Dry tap" on bone marrow biopsy
  - Hairy cells induce marrow fibrosis
- Tartrate-resistant acid phosphatase (TRAP)
  - Cellular enzyme
  - Hairy cells: strong positivity for TRAP staining

Spleen

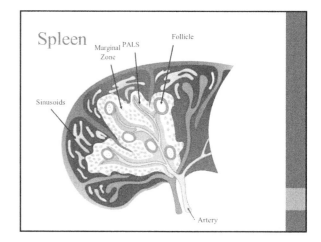

Hairy Cell Leukemia
Clinical features

- Median age: 52
- Presenting feature often abdominal pain
- Fatigue, weakness
- Splenomegaly
- Bone marrow suppression (anemia, ↓platelets)

Cladribine
2-chlorodeoxyadenosine (2-CdA)

- Preferred initial therapy for HCL
- Excellent clinical response
- Similar to adenosine ("purine analog")
- Highly toxic to leukemic cells in HCL

Cladribine   Deoxyadenosine

Hodgkin Lymphoma

Jason Ryan, MD, MPH

Lymphomas

- Malignancies of lymphocytes (B cells, T cells)
- Often involve lymph nodes
- Also "extranodal" (skin, GI tract)

Wikipedia/Public Domain

Lymphomas
Signs and Symptoms

- Enlarged, painless lymph nodes
- "B symptoms"
  - Systemic symptoms
  - Fever, chills, night sweats

Lymphomas

Tissue
Biopsy

↓

Malignant Lymphocytes

↓

Reed-Sternberg
Cells?

No / \ Yes

Non-Hodgkin   Hodgkin
Lymphoma   Lymphoma

Reed-Sternberg Cells

- Large cell
- Multi-lobed nucleus
  - Two halves; often mirror images ("owl-eyed")
- Usually derive from B cells (rarely from T cells)
- Usually CD15+ and CD30+
- Usually NOT positive for B cell markers
  - CD19, CD20, CD21, CD22
- Sometimes seen in other disorders

Reed-Sternberg Cells

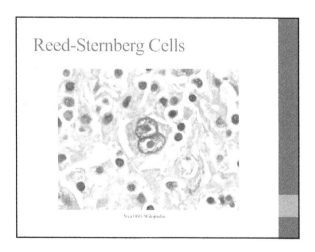

Nxa1991/Wikipedia

Hodgkin Lymphoma

- Malignant cell: Reed-Sternberg cell
  - A minority of cells in enlarged nodes (~1 to 5%)
- Release cytokines ☐ generate reactive cells
  - Majority of cells in node are reactive
  - B symptoms common (more than non-Hodgkin lymphoma)
  - Macrophages may activate ☐ hypercalcemia

$$25\text{-OH Vitamin D} \xrightarrow{1\alpha \text{ - hydroxylase}} 1,25\text{-OH}_2 \text{ Vitamin D}$$

Hodgkin Lymphoma

- Commonly presents with cervical lymphadenopathy
  - Often with B symptoms
- Spreads in a very predictable manner
- Limited disease highly curable
- Stage is strongest predictor of prognosis

Hodgkin Lymphoma

- Bimodal age distribution
  - Peaks at age 20 and 65
- Risk factors
  - Prior EBV infection (virus infects B cells)
  - Immunosuppression (HIV, transplant)
  - Autoimmune disease: Rheumatoid arthritis and lupus
- Treatment: chemotherapy and radiation

Classification

Hodgkin Lymphoma

Classical (cellular background)

Nodular lymphocyte predominant

Nodular Sclerosing — Mixed Cellularity — Lymphocyte Rich — Lymphocyte Depleted

Lymphocyte Predominant

Nodular Lymphocyte Predominant

- Rare variant of Hodgkin lymphoma
- Malignant cell: LP cells
  - Lymphocyte predominant
  - Sometimes called "popcorn cells"
- Unusual surface marker expression
  - Usually lack CD15 and CD30
  - Express CD20

Popcorn Cells

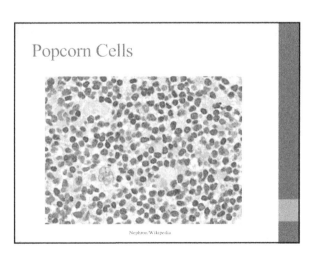

Nephron/Wikipedia

100

Classical Hodgkin Lymphoma

- Nodular sclerosing
  - Most common type HL: 60% to 80% of all cases
  - More common in women (most HL more common men)
  - Often presents with a mediastinal mass on CXR
  - Reed-Sternberg cells seen in clear space ("lacunar variant")
  - Slow growing ("indolent")
  - Good long-term survival

Classical Hodgkin Lymphoma

- Mixed cellularity
  - Eosinophils, neutrophils, macrophages, plasma cells
- Lymphocyte rich
  - Excellent prognosis
- Lymphocyte depleted
  - Poor prognosis

Hodgkin versus. Non-Hodgkin
Clinical Features

Hodgkin	Non-Hodgkin
- Often localized	- Often multiple peripheral sites
- Orderly spread from node to node	- Noncontiguous spread
- Extranodal involvement rare	- Extranodal involvement common
	- GI (thickened bowel wall)
	- Skin

Hodgkin Lymphoma
Treatment

- Many different regimens
- ABVD
  - Adriamycin (doxorubicin) - cytotoxic antibiotics
  - Bleomycin - cytotoxic antibiotics
  - Vinblastine – microtubule inhibitor
  - Dacarbazine – alkylating agent

Non-Hodgkin Lymphoma

Jason Ryan, MD, MPH

Lymphomas

- Malignancies of lymphocytes (B cells, T cells)
- Often involve lymph nodes
- Also "extranodal" (skin, GI tract)

Wikipedia/Public Domain

Lymphomas

Tissue
Biopsy
↓
Malignant Lymphocytes
↓
Reed-Sternberg
Cells?

No / \ Yes

Non-Hodgkin   Hodgkin
Lymphoma   Lymphoma

Hodgkin versus. Non-Hodgkin
Clinical Features

Hodgkin	Non-Hodgkin
- Often localized	- Often multiple peripheral sites
- Orderly spread from node to node	- Noncontiguous spread
- Extranodal involvement rare	- Extranodal involvement common
	- GI (thickened bowel wall)
	- Skin

Waldeyer's Ring

- Lymphoid tissue in the pharynx
- Often involved in non-Hodgkin lymphoma
  - Rare in Hodgkin lymphoma

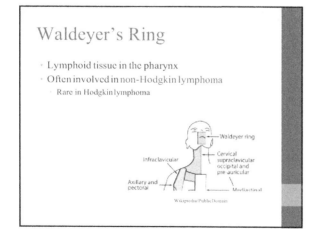

Wikipedia/Public Domain

Lymphocyte Antigens

Primarily T-Cell Associated	Primarily B-cell Associated
CD1	CD10
CD2	CD19
CD3	CD20
CD4	CD21
CD5	CD22
CD7	CD23
CD8	

Non-Hodgkin Lymphoma

- B and T cell malignancies
  - Most are B cell disorders
  - Malignant cells obliterate lymph node architecture
- More than two dozen subtypes per WHO
- Classified by:
  - B versus T cell
  - Cell size (small versus large)
  - Histologic appearance
  - Expression of markers ("immunophenotype")
  - Genetics

Non-Hodgkin Lymphoma

- Follicular
- Marginal cell
- Mantle zone
- Diffuse Large B Cell
- Small lymphocytic lymphoma
- Burkitt's
- Adult T-cell Leukemia/Lymphoma
- Cutaneous T-cell Lymphomas

Lymph Nodes

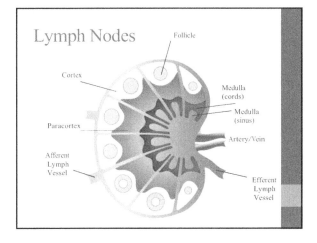

Lymphoid Follicles

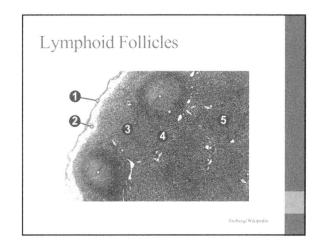

Gleiberg/Wikipedia

Diffuse Large B-cell Lymphoma

- Most common NH lymphoma
- B cell malignancy
  - Express CD19, CD20
  - Most cells express surface immunoglobulin

Diffuse Large B-cell Lymphoma

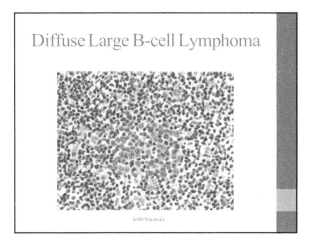

KGH/Wikipedia

Diffuse Large B-cell Lymphoma

- Median age at presentation is 64 years
- Occurs in HIV
  - AIDS defining malignancy

Diffuse Large B-cell Lymphoma
Prognosis

- Variable prognosis
- International Prognostic Index (IPI) score
  - Age >60 years
  - Increased LDH
  - Patient functional status
  - Clinical stage
  - Number of extranodal sites

Rituximab

- Monoclonal CD20 antibody
- Used in CD20+ B cell lymphomas
  - Diffuse large B cell
  - Follicular

Follicular Lymphoma

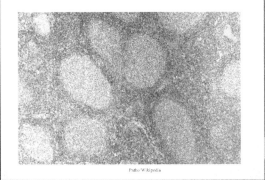

Patho Wikipedia

Follicular Lymphoma

- B cell malignancy
  - Usually express CD19, CD20
  - Most cells express surface immunoglobulin

Follicular Lymphoma

- Genetic hallmark: 14;18 translocation
- Overexpression of BCL2
  - Blocks apoptosis ("antagonist" of apoptosis)
  - Germinal center B cells usually lack BCL2
  - Undergo apoptosis unless selected by somatic hypermutation

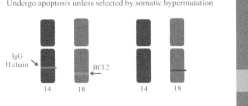

Follicular Lymphoma

- Median age at diagnosis: 65 years
- Indolent course: waxes/wanes for years
  - Not all patients require treatment
  - Difficult to cure
- Diffuse large B cell lymphoma (DLBCL)
  - Histologic transformation: 10 to 70% cases over time
  - Poor prognosis

Lymphoma vs. Reactive

- Follicular lymphoma vs. reactive lymphadenopathy
  - Both have ↑ follicle growth
  - Must distinguish in diagnosis of lymphoma
- Reactive lymphadenopathy (LAD)
  - Somatic hypermutation of B cells
  - Apoptosis of many B cells
  - B cell death ⁓ debris ⁓ macrophages

Lymphoma vs. Reactive

Lymphoma	Reactive LAD
Similar size/shape follicles	Varying size/shape follicles
Relative absence of macrophages	Tingible body (debris-laden) macrophages
++ BCL2 Staining	-- BCL2 Staining

Mantle Cell Lymphoma

- B cell malignancy
  - Follicle mantle or germinal center
  - Usually express CD19, CD20
  - Most cells express surface immunoglobulin
  - Express CD5 ("Co-express CD20 and CD5")
- Median age at diagnosis: 68 years
- Median overall survival: 3 to 4 years (poor prognosis)

Mantle Cell Lymphoma

- 50 to 65%: 11:14 translocation
- Overexpression of cyclin D1
  - Promotes cell cycle transition from G1 to S phase

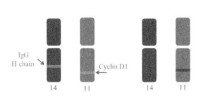

Marginal Zone Lymphoma

- B cell malignancies
- Marginal zone forms from inflammation
- Often extranodal
- Lymphoma in chronic inflammatory disorders
  - Salivary glands in Sjogren's
  - Thyroid gland in Hashimoto's thyroiditis
  - Stomach in chronic H. Pylori infection (MAL Toma)

Small Lymphocytic Lymphoma

- CD5+ B cells
  - "Co-express CD20 and CD5"
  - Similar markers to mantle cell lymphoma
  - Typically negative for cyclin D1
- Same malignant cells as CLL
  - Only difference is degree of lymphocytosis (↑WBC)
  - Peripheral blood: normal or mild lymphocytosis
- SLL definition: lymphocyte count of <5000
  - If >5000 ☐ CLL

Burkitt's Lymphoma

- B cell malignancy
  - Usually express CD19, CD20
  - Most cells express surface immunoglobulin
- Very aggressive – rapid proliferation
- Key distinctions:
  - "Starry sky" morphology
  - Epstein-Barr virus (EBV)
  - C-myc translocation

Burkitt's Lymphoma

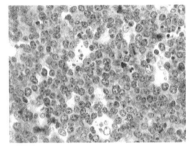

Wikipedia/Public Domain

Burkitt's Lymphoma

- Endemic form
  - Found in Africa and New Guinea
  - 30 to 50% of childhood cancer in some regions
  - Children four to seven years old
  - Male to female ratio ~ 2:1
  - Commonly presents as mass in the mandible
- Sporadic form
  - Also occurs in children
  - Abdominal mass: ileocecum or peritoneum

Burkitt's Lymphoma

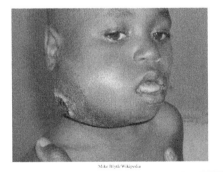

Mike Blyth/Wikipedia

Burkitt's Lymphoma
Associations

- Epstein Barr virus (EBV) infection
  - Nearly all endemic tumors associated with latent infection
  - Express CD21 (EBV receptor)

Burkitt's Lymphoma
Associations

- C-myc translocation
  - Growth promoter
  - Activates transcription

IgG
H chain

C-myc

14   8   14   8

T-C ell Leukemia/Lymphoma

- CD4+ T cell malignancy
- Occurs with HTLV-1 infection
  - RNA Virus
  - Infects CD4+ T cells
- Key diagnostic test: anti-HTLV1 antibodies

T-C ell Leukemia/Lymphoma

- Clinical scenario
  - Patient from Japan, Caribbean, West Africa (endemic regions)
  - Lymphocytosis
  - Lymphadenopathy
  - Skin lesions (ulcers, nodules, papular rash)
  - Rapidly progressive symptoms — usually fatal in months
- Lytic bone lesions with ↑ calcium
  - Don't confuse with multiple myeloma

Cutaneous T-cell Lymphoma
CTCL

- Skin disorder of malignant T-cells
  - Variable expression of CD markers
- Presents with skin lesions
  - Localized disease: Mycosis Fungoides
  - Diffuse systemic disease: Sezary syndrome

Cutaneous T-cell Lymphoma
CTCL

- Mycosis Fungoides
  - Patches, plaques, tumors
  - Varying size/shape
  - Lesions progress slowly changing size/shape/appearance
  - "Indolent": Slowly developing
  - Classically in a "bathing trunk" distribution
- Diagnosis: Skin biopsy shows lymphoid cells
  - Upper dermis
  - Epidermal aggregates (Pautrier microabscesses)

Cutaneous T-cell Lymphoma
CTCL

- Sezary syndrome
  - T-cell lymphoma affecting skin of entire body
  - Widespread erythema (skin bright red)
  - Lymphadenopathy
  - Malignant cells in blood (Sezary cells)

Multi-lobed nucleus
"Cerebriform"

El*Falaf

Plasma Cell Disorders

Jason Ryan, MD, MPH

Hematopoiesis

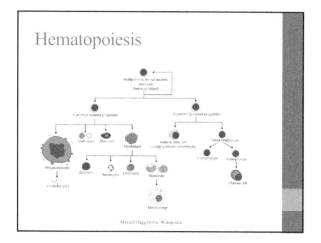

Mikael Häggström /Wikipedia

Multiple Myeloma

- Malignancy of plasma cells
  - Dependent on IL-6
  - Required for myeloma cell proliferation
- Excess production of immunoglobulin
- Disorder of older patients (median age: 66)

IL-6

Multiple Myeloma

- IgG (~50%)
- IgA (~20%)
- Light chains only (~15%)
- "Paraproteins"

IgG   IgA

Light   Light

Heavy   Heavy

Fvasconcellos /Wikipedia

Martin Brändli /Wikipedia

Light Chains

- Two types: Kappa (κ) or lambda (λ)
  - Each antibody: two identical light chains
  - Heavy chain type determines antibody type: G, A, E, etc.
- Slight excess of light chains produced normally
- Filtered by glomerulus ☐ reabsorbed proximal tubule

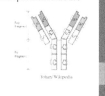

Johan/Wikipedia

Light Chains

- Excess light chains can occur in multiple myeloma
- Excess light chains leads to pathology:
  - Renal damage
  - AL amyloidosis

Johan/Wikipedia

SPEP
Serum protein electrophoresis

- Electrical current separates serum proteins
  - Based on size and charge
- Gamma fraction contains immunoglobulin
- Multiple myeloma: "M spike"

Normal SPEP   Multiple Myeloma

Steven Fruitsmaak

Multiple Myeloma
Clinical Features

- Bone pain/fractures
- Hypercalcemia
- Renal failure
- Anemia
- Infections

Multiple Myeloma
Bone/hypercalcemia

- Osteoclast-mediated bone resorption
- Caused by cytokines from myeloma cells
- "Lytic lesions" on x-ray ("punched out")
- Pathologic fractures, especially vertebral column
- Elevated serum calcium

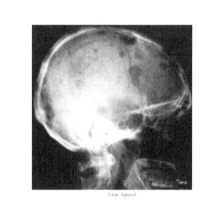

Utsav Agrawal

Multiple Myeloma
Renal Failure

- Caused by light chains and hypercalcemia
- Light chains ("myeloma kidney")
  - Small amount of light chains normally filtered/reabsorbed
  - MM: proximal tubular capacity exceeded
  - Light chains reach distal tubule
  - Combine with Tamm–Horsfall mucoprotein (THP)
  - Form obstructing casts
  - Light chains in urine = "Bence Jones" proteins

Multiple Myeloma
Renal Failure

- Hypercalcemia
  - Impairs renal ability to concentrate urine
  - Polyuria → volume contraction
  - Decreased GFR

Multiple Myeloma
Renal Failure

- Urine dipstick negative for protein
  - Mostly detects albumin
  - Poor detection of light chains
- Urine protein electrophoresis (UPEP)
  - Similar to SPEP ("SPEP/UPEP")
  - Detects light chains ("Bence Jones proteins")

J3D3

Multiple Myeloma
Renal Failure

- Serum free light chain
  - Antibody-based system
  - Sensitive test for serum kappa/lambda light chains
  - Alternative to UPEP

Multiple Myeloma
Anemia

- Normocytic, normochromic
- Multifactorial
  - Bone marrow replacement by plasma cells
  - Renal failure (low EPO)
- Weakness, pallor often present at diagnosis

Multiple Myeloma
Infections

- Infection is leading cause of death
- Decreased production of normal immunoglobulins
  - Depressed humoral immunity
- Recurrent bacterial infections
  - Strep Pneumoniae
  - Staph Aureus
  - E. Coli

Rouleaux

- RBCs form a stack of coins
- Caused by elevated protein levels in plasma

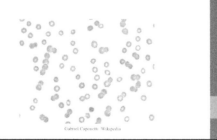

Gabriel Caponetti Wikipedia

Multiple Myeloma
Diagnosis

- SPEP: Monoclonal protein
- Diagnostic criteria
  - Bone marrow biopsy: clonal bone marrow plasma cells
  - End-organ damage

MGUS
Monoclonal gammopathy of undetermined significance

- Asymptomatic plasma cell disorder
- Abnormal SPEP (presence of M protein)
- No end-organ damage
- Can progress to multiple myeloma
- Often detected in workup of another problem
  - Anemia
  - Hypercalcemia
  - Bone pain

Waldenstrom Macroglobulinemia

- Also called lymphoplasmacytic lymphoma
- B-cell lymphoma
- Tumor cells differentiate into plasma cells
- Produce IgM antibodies
- Leads to hyperviscosity symptoms

Martin Brändli-Wikipedia

Waldenstrom Macroglobulinemia

- Weakness, fatigue, weight loss
- Lymphadenopathy (25% of patients)
  - Sometimes splenomegaly, hepatomegaly
- No osteolytic bone lesions
- SPEP: M spike from IgM

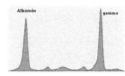

Steven Fruitsmaak

Hyperviscosity Syndrome

- IgM increases viscosity of blood
- Sluggish blood flow and sludging
- CNS: Headache, dizziness, coma
- Visual impairment
- Medical emergency: emergent plasmapheresis

Poiseuille's Law	
R =	$\dfrac{8\,\eta\ (viscosity)\ L\ (length)}{\Pi\ r\ (radius)^4}$

Amyloidosis

Jason Ryan, MD, MPH

Amyloid

- Amyloid: Pathologic aggregate of amyloid proteins
- "Pathologic:" Damages tissues
- Accumulates in extracellular space of tissues
- Amyloid proteins:
  - More than 20 proteins form amyloid
  - Different proteins = different diseases

Amyloid

- Localized amyloid deposition
  - Alzheimer's: Beta Amyloid
  - Cerebral amyloid angiopathy: Beta Amyloid
  - Type II diabetes: Amylin deposits in pancreas
- Diffuse amyloid deposition = amyloidosis

Systemic Amyloidosis

- Primary (AL) amyloidosis: Light chains
- Secondary (AA) amyloidosis: Serum amyloid A
- Dialysis-related amyloidosis: Beta-2 microglobulin
- Age-related systemic amyloidosis: : Transthyretin
- Familial
  - Many types
  - Most common: Abnormal transthyretin gene

Transthyretin

- Formerly called prealbumin
- Transports thyroid hormone and retinol (vitamin A)
- Amyloidosis: Amyloid transthyretin (ATTR)
- Mutant form seen in hereditary amyloidosis
- Normal transthyretin seen in age-related amyloidosis

Amyloid

- Pink on standard biopsy
  - Similar to collagen, fibrin, other proteins
- Specialized stain for detection
  - Congo red
  - Pink under ordinary light
  - Shows apple-green birefringence under polarized light

Ed Uthman, MD

Amyloid

- Forms beta-pleated sheets
  - Secondary protein structure
  - Detected by crystallography and spectroscopy
- Responsible for Congo Red staining

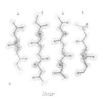

Darryl

AL Amyloidosis
Primary Amyloidosis

- Plasma cell malignancy ("dyscrasia")
  - Amyloid formed from light chains
  - Can occur alone
  - Also in association with MM, Waldenstrom's, lymphoma
- Bone marrow biopsy: monoclonal plasma cells
- Can be treated with stem cell transplantation

AA Amyloidosis
Secondary Amyloidosis

- Occurs in chronic inflammatory conditions
- Rheumatoid arthritis, ankylosing spondylitis, IBD
- Amyloid: serum amyloid A (SAA) proteins
  - SAA proteins: acute phase reactants
  - Apolipoproteins
  - Many roles in inflammatory response

Familial Mediterranean Fever

- Rare hereditary disorder
- Inflammatory disease
- Involves neutrophils
- Recurrent episodes of fever and inflammatory pain
- "Serosal" inflammation
  - Abdominal pain; pericarditis
- Secondary (AA) amyloidosis: major cause of death
- Treatment: Colchicine (inhibits neutrohpils)

Neutrophil

Mikael Häggström

Dialysis-related Amyloidosis

- β2 microglobulin
- Complication of renal failure
- Dialysis does not effectively remove β2 microglobulin
- Bones, joints, tendons
- Shoulder pain
- Carpal tunnel syndrome

MHC I

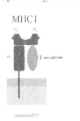

atropos235

Age-related Amyloidosis
Senile Amyloidosis

- Wild-type (normal) transthyretin
- Usually develops >70 years old
- Predominantly occurs in the heart
- Rarely other significant organ involvement

Familial Amyloidosis

- Mutant transthyretin
- Produced by liver
- Can be treated with liver transplant
- Symptoms in adulthood

Wikipedia/Public Domain

Amyloidosis
Clinical Features

- May involve almost any tissue/organ
- Skin: Periorbital purpura (raccoon eyes)
- Muscles: Enlarged tongue
- Nerves: Peripheral neuropathy
- Liver: Hepatomegaly
- Bowel: Malabsorption
- Blood vessels: Bleeding

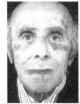

Professor P N Hawkins

Amyloidosis
Clinical Features

- Kidneys
  - Most commonly involved organ
  - Leads to proteinuria and the nephrotic syndrome

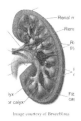

Image courtesy of BruceBlaus

Amyloidosis
Clinical Features

- Heart
  - Can cause a restrictive cardiomyopathy
  - Common with light chains and transthyretin amyloidosis
  - Increased wall thickness, diastolic heart failure
  - Arrhythmias, sudden death

 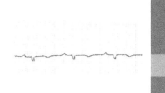

Amyloidosis
Diagnosis

- Biopsy: tissue infiltration of amyloid
- Abdominal fat pad preferred
  - Easy to access (low risk procedure)
  - Good sensitivity

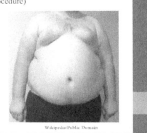

Wikipedia/Public Domain

Amyloidosis

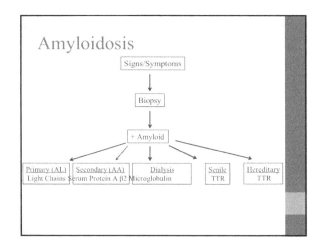

114

Myeloproliferative Disorders

Jason Ryan, MD, MPH

Myeloproliferative Disorders

- Disorders of myeloid proliferation
  - Granulocytes, red cells, platelets
- Often leads to increased peripheral cell counts
  - Chronic myeloid leukemia: granulocytes
  - Essential thrombocytosis: platelets
  - Polycythemia vera: red blood cells

Myeloproliferative Disorders
Major Types

- Chronic myeloid leukemia (granulocytes)
- Essential thrombocytosis (platelets)
- Polycythemia vera (red blood cells)
- Myelofibrosis

Myeloproliferative Disorders
Major Types

- Chronic myeloid leukemia (granulocytes)
- Essential thrombocytosis (platelets)
- Polycythemia vera (red blood cells)
- Myelofibrosis

Myeloproliferative Disorders
Major Types

Disorder	Genetics
Chronic Myelogenous Leukemia	Philadelphia Chromosome t 9;22; BCR-ABL
Polycythemia Vera	JAK2 (~100%)
Essential Thrombocytosis	JAK2 (~60%)
Myelofibrosis	JAK2 (~60%)

JAK2 Mutation

- Gene for cytoplasmic tyrosine kinase
  - Chromosome 9
- Mutation ☐ ↑ tyrosine phosphorylation
- Progenitor cells: Hypersensitivity to cytokines
- More growth; longer survival

Polycythemia Vera

- Elevated red blood cell mass

Measurement	Normal	P. Vera
Hgb (g/dL)	15	20
Hct (%)	45	60

Polycythemia Vera

- Must exclude other causes
  - Hypoxia (lung disease)
  - EPO secreting tumor (renal cell carcinoma)

Measurement	Hypoxia	RCC	P. Vera
PaO$_2$	↓	Normal	Normal
EPO	↑	↑	↓

Polycythemia Vera
Symptom Mechanisms

- Increased RBC mass
  - Leads to increase in blood volume
  - Causes hypertension, flushing
- Thrombosis
  - Increased viscosity of blood
  - Also increased platelets

$$ \text{Poiseuille's Law} $$
$$ R = \frac{8\,\eta\,(\text{viscosity})\;L\,(\text{length})}{\Pi\,r\,(\text{radius})^4} $$

Polycythemia Vera
Symptoms

- Many patients asymptomatic (routine CBC)
- Red, puffy skin ("facial plethora")
- Aquagenic pruritus
  - "Unbearable" pruritus after warm bath or shower
- Deep vein thrombosis
  - Classically Budd Chiari syndrome (hepatic vein)

Polycythemia Vera
Treatment

- Phlebotomy
- Hydroxyurea
  - Inhibits ribonucleotide reductase
  - Blocks formation of deoxynucleotides for DNA

Public Domain

Polycythemia Vera
Complications

- Spent phase (~15% of patients)
  - Progression to myelofibrosis
- Leukemia
  - Usually acute myeloid leukemia (AML)
  - Rarely chronic myeloid leukemia (CML)
- Gout
  - Excess DNA turnover from ↑ RBC production
  - Increased purine metabolism ☐ ↑ uric acid
  - Also seen in CML

Essential thrombocytosis
Essential thrombocythemia

- Malignant proliferation of myeloid cells
- Predominantly affects megakaryocytes/platelets

Essential thrombocytosis
Essential thrombocythemia

- "Diagnosis of exclusion"
- Must exclude a reactive thrombocytosis
  - Iron deficiency anemia
  - Acute bleeding or hemolysis
  - Infections/inflammation
  - Metastatic cancer
- Key blood test: acute phase reactants
  - C-reactive protein, fibrinogen, ESR, ferritin
  - Increased levels suggest occult inflammatory process

Essential thrombocytosis
Symptoms

- Abnormal platelet function
- Bleeding
- Thrombosis

Essential thrombocytosis
Prognosis and Treatment

- Most patients have no disease-related complications
- Polycythemia vera complications unusual
  - AML, myelofibrosis, hyperuricemia
- High risk patients treated with:
  - Hydroxyurea
  - Aspirin

Myelofibrosis

- Primary myelofibrosis
  - Myeloproliferative disorder
- Secondary myelofibrosis
  - Polycythemia vera, chronic leukemia, other causes

Primary Myelofibrosis

- Excess collagen from fibroblasts ⊐ marrow fibrosis
- Stimulation by growth factors of megakaryocytes
  - Platelet-derived growth factor (PDGF)
  - Transforming growth factor beta (TGF-B)

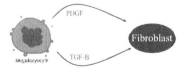

Primary Myelofibrosis
Pathophysiology

- Marrow failure □ extramedullary hematopoiesis
- Spleen, liver, lymph nodes
- Can be seen in CNS, lungs, bladder, even in skin!

Primary Myelofibrosis
Clinical Features

- Occurs in older patients (median age 67)
- Fatigue, weight loss, night sweats
  - Increased metabolism

Primary Myelofibrosis
Clinical Features

- Massive splenomegaly
  - Spleen: principle site of extramedullary hematopoiesis
  - Left upper abdominal pain
  - Early satiety (compression of stomach)
- May also see enlarged liver, lymph nodes
- Leukoerythroblastosis
  - Inappropriate release of cells from marrow
  - Immature erythroid and granulocyte precursors in blood

Primary Myelofibrosis
Clinical Features

- Normocytic, normochromic anemia
  - Severe
  - Hemoglobin often less than 10g/dL
- WBC and platelets variable
  - Elevated, normal, or reduced
  - Immature neutrophils seen
  - Myeloblasts
- Hyperuricemia (gout)
  - High cell turnover □ increased metabolism
- Treatment: Stem cell transplant

Tear Drop Cells
Dacrocytes

- Classic finding of myelofibrosis
- Red blood cells deformed leaving fibrotic marrow

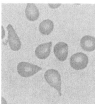

Paulo Henrique Orlandi Mourao/Wikipedia

Langerhans Cell Histiocytosis

- Histiocyte = connective tissue macrophage
- Histiocytosis = proliferation of histiocytes
- Langerhans Cell = dendritic cells
  - Common in skin, connective tissue
  - Consume antigens
  - Migrate to lymph nodes
  - Present antigens □ activate T-cells

Langerhans Cell Histiocytosis

- Clonal proliferation of dendritic cells
- Cells of myeloid origin
- Express CD1a, S100, CD207
    - Same as Langerhans cells

Birbeck Granules

- Found in cytoplasm of Langerhans cells
- Seen on electron microscopy

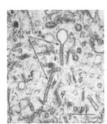

Yale Rose/Wikipedia

Langerhans Cell Histiocytosis
Clinical Features

- Most common in children
- Can involve any organ system
- Often involves bone and skin

Langerhans Cell Histiocytosis
Clinical Features

Letterer-Siwe Disease		Eosinophilic Granuloma
Occurs in child (~2 years old) Diffuse skin rash Cystic bone lesions Multi-system failure Rapidly fatal	Spectrum	Adolescents No skin involvement Pathologic bone fracture NOT osteosarcoma Langerhans cells/eosinophils

Hand-Schuller-Christian Disease
Triad: skull, diabetes insipidus, exophthalmos
Scalp lesion
Posterior pituitary (DI)
Protrusion of eye

Langerhans Cell Histiocytosis
Clinical Features

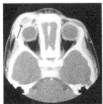 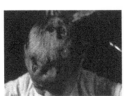

Madhero88/Wikipedia

Coastline/Wikipedia

Antimetabolites

Jason Ryan, MD, MPH

Antimetabolites

- Chemotherapy drugs used to treat malignancy
- Block formation of components of DNA
- Cell cycle specific
- Toxic effects in S phase of cell cycle

Antimetabolites

- Cytarabine
- Cladribine
- Methotrexate
- 5-fluorouracil
- Azathioprine
- 6-mercaptopurine
- 6-thioguanine
- Hydroxyurea

Nitrogenous Bases

Pyrimidines

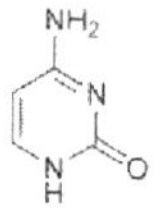

Cytosine 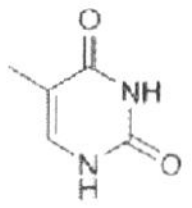   Thymine 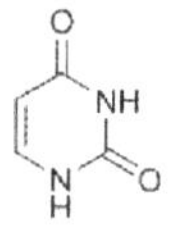   Uracil

Purines

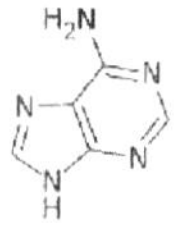

Adenine 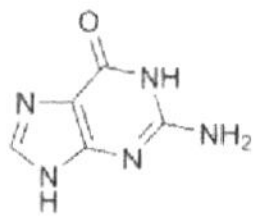   Guanine

---

Nucleotides

Pyrimidines

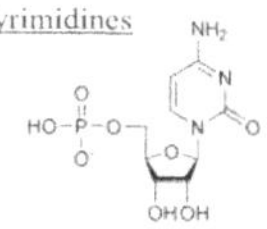

Cytidine 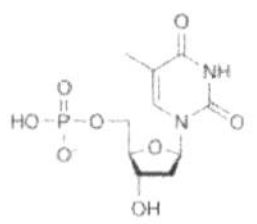   Thymidine 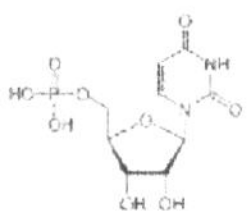   Uridine

Purines

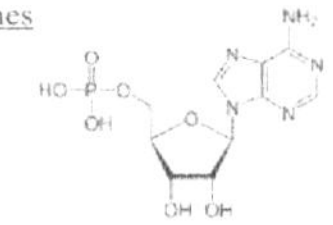

Adenosine 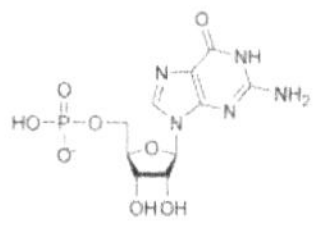   Guanosine

---

Deoxyribonucleotides

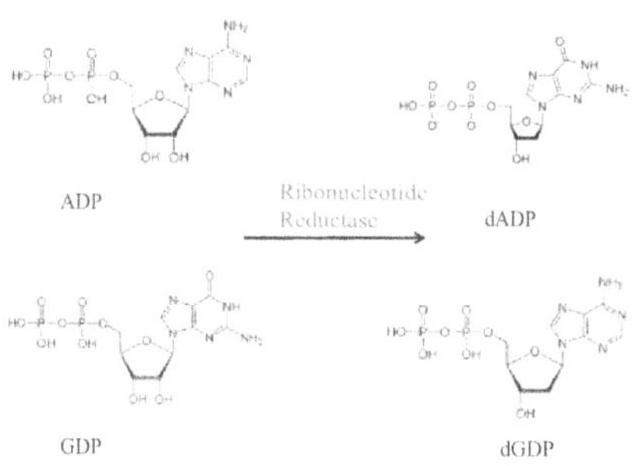

ADP   Ribonucleotide Reductase   dADP

GDP   dGDP

Common Side Effects

- Drugs target rapidly dividing cells (DNA synthesis)
- Bone marrow precursors cells: rapidly dividing
- Myelosuppression
  - Megaloblastic anemia
  - Thrombocytopenia
  - Leukopenia
- Absolute neutrophil count (ANC)
  - Less than 500 cells/μL = neutropenia
  - High risk of infections

Megaloblastic Anemia

- Anemia ($\downarrow$Hct)
- Large RBCs ($\uparrow$MCV)
- Hypersegmented neutrophils
- Commonly caused by defective DNA production
  - B12/Folate deficiency
  - Chemotherapy drugs (MTX, 5-FU, hydroxyurea)

Wikipedia:Public Domain

Cytarabine
Ara-C or cytosine arabinoside

- Pyrimidine analog
- Mimics cytidine
- Inhibits DNA polymerase

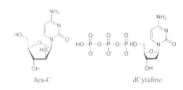

Ara-C   dCytidine

Cytarabine
Ara-C or cytosine arabinoside

- Only effective in leukemia and lymphomas
- Adverse effects
  - Myelosuppression
  - Nausea/vomiting
  - High doses: Neurotoxicity
  - Peripheral neuropathy, confusion, cerebellar ataxia

Cladribine

- Purine analog
- Mimics adenosine
- Highly toxic to lymphocytes
- Drug of choice in hairy cell leukemia
- Main adverse effect is myelosuppression

Adenosine   Cladribine

Methotrexate

- Mimics of folate
- Inhibits dihydrofolate reductase
- Blocks synthesis if tetrahydrofolate
- Required for DNA, RNA, some proteins
- Blocks synthesis thymidine (dTMP)

Folate   Methotrexate

Thymidine

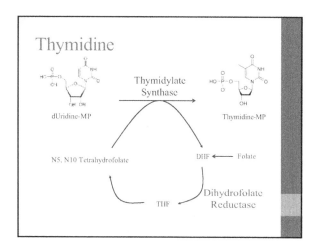

dUridine-MP → Thymidine-MP

Thymidylate Synthase

N5, N10 Tetrahydrofolate

DHF ← Folate

THF

Dihydrofolate Reductase

Methotrexate
Clinical Uses

- Oral or intravenous
- Many malignancies
  - Solid tumors
  - Leukemia/Lymphomas
- Immunosuppression
  - Autoimmune diseases
  - "Steroid sparing" agents
  - Used to wean/eliminate need for long-term steroid use
- Pregnancy abortion
  - Ectopic/tubal pregnancies

Methotrexate
Side Effects

- Myelosuppression
  - More common with high doses
  - Reversible with leucovorin (folinic acid)
  - Converted to THF
  - Does not require dihydrofolate reductase
  - "Leucovorin rescue"

Methotrexate
Side Effects

- Mucositis (mouth soreness)
  - Occurs with many chemo agents
  - Common with methotrexate
  - GI epithelial cell damage
  - Loss of mucosal integrity ⁻ pain, bacterial growth
- Abnormal LFTs, GI upset

Methotrexate
Side Effects

- Rarely causes methotrexate-induced lung injury
  - Often after week/months of low-dose therapy
  - Usually a hypersensitivity reaction
  - Lymphocytes, eosinophils
  - Can progress to pulmonary fibrosis
  - Usually resolves on discontinuation of drug

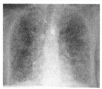

5-Fluorouracil
5-FU

Fluorouracil   Uracil

- Mimics uracil (pyrimidine)
- Converted to 5-FdUMP (abnormal dUMP)
- Inhibition thymidylate synthase
- Blocks dTMP synthesis ("thymineless death")
- Effects enhanced by leucovorin

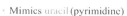

5-Fluorouracil

5-FU

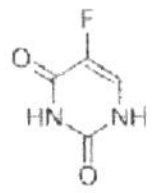

Fluorouracil

- Commonly used in colorectal cancer
- Other solid tumors: breast, pancreas
- Topical therapy for basal cell skin cancer
- Adverse effects
  - Myelosuppression
  - Nausea/vomiting/diarrhea
  - Mucositis
  - Cerebellar ataxia and encephalopathy (rare)
  - Coronary vasospasm

6- Mercaptopurine

- Mimics hypoxanthine/guanine (purines)
- Added to PRPP by HGPRT ☐ Thioinosinic acid
- Inhibits multiple steps in purine salvage
- ↓IMP/AMP/GMP

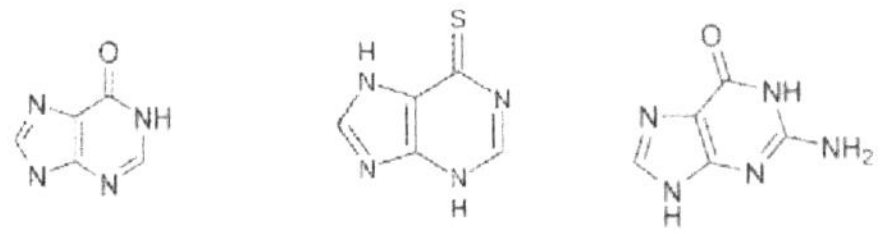

Hypoxanthine   6-MP   Guanine

6-Mercaptopurine

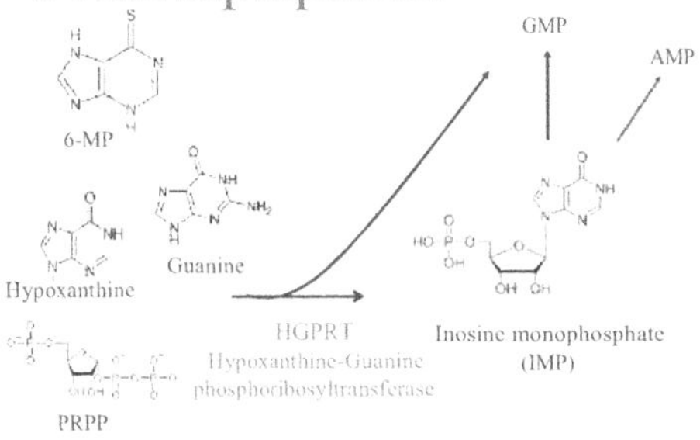

Purine Salvage Pathway

Azathioprine

- Pro-drug
- Converted by the body to 6-MP

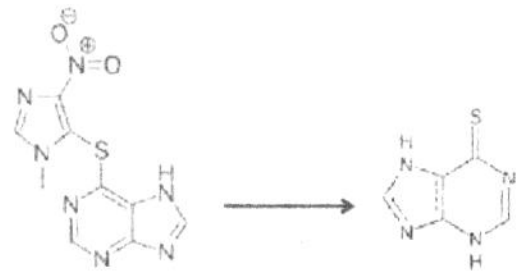

Azathioprine   6-MP

Azathioprine/6-MP

Clinical Uses

- Immunosuppression
  - Steroid sparing agents
  - Inflammatory bowel disease
  - Solid organ transplant
  - Autoimmune diseases

Azathioprine/6-MP

Adverse Effects

- Myelosuppression
- Abnormal LFTs
- Anorexia/nausea/vomiting

123

Xanthine Oxidase

- Purine metabolism enzyme
- Converts xanthine into uric acid
- Inhibited by allopurinol and febuxostat (gout)

Azathioprine/6-MP

- Also metabolized by xanthine oxidase
- Converts 6-MP to inactive metabolite
- Caution with allopurinol/febuxostat

6- Thioguanine

- Also mimics hypoxanthine/guanine (purines)
- Similar mechanism to 6-MP
- ↓IMP/AMP/GMP

Hydroxyurea

- Inhibits ribonucleotide reductase
- Blocks formation of deoxynucleotides
- Good oral bioavailability – can be used PO
- Main adverse effect is myelosuppression

Hydroxyurea

- Rarely used for malignancy
- Used for polycythemia vera, essential thrombocytosis
- Used in sickle cell anemia
  - Increases fetal hemoglobin levels (mechanism unclear)

Antimetabolites

Folate	Purines	Pyrimidines	Other
Methotrexate	Cladribine 6-MP Azathioprine 6-TG	Cytarabine 5-FU	Hydroxyurea

Alkylating Agents

Jason Ryan, MD, MPH

Alkyl Groups

- Molecular groups with formula: C_nH_{2n+1}
- Methyl group: $-CH_3$
- Ethyl group: $-CH_2CH_3$
- Propyl group: $-CH_2CH_2CH_3$

Alkylating Agents

- Add alkyl groups to nucleotide bases
- Most commonly N7 nitrogen of guanine
- DNA strands cross link
- Inhibit DNA replication and cause DNA damage
- Cell cycle non-specific

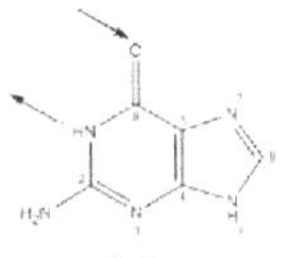

Guanine

Alkylating Agents

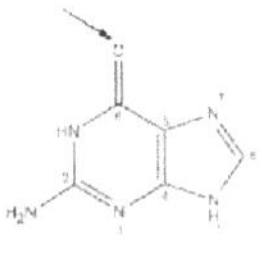

Guanine

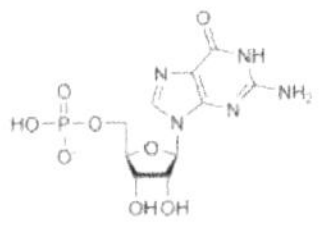

Guanosine

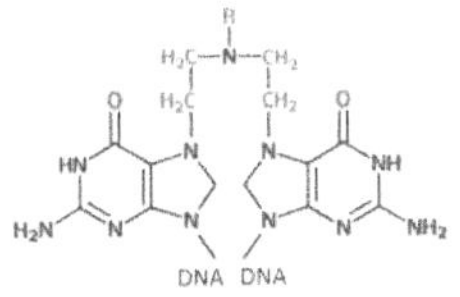

N7 interstrand crosslinked DNA

Alkylating Agents

- Nitrogen mustards
- Nitrosoureas
- Busulfan
- Dacarbazine

Nitrogen Mustards
Alkylating Agents

- Alkylating agents similar to mustard gas
- Contain nitrogen and two chlorine atoms

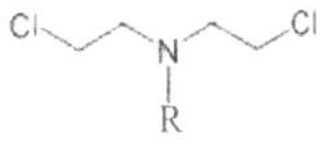

Nitrogen Mustards
Alkylating Agents

Mechlorethamine

Cyclophosphamide

Melphalan

Chlorambucil

Ifosfamide

Cyclophosphamide

- Intravenous or oral forms
  - Good bioavailability when given orally
- Powerful immunosuppressant
  - Used in vasculitis, glomerulonephritis (oral)
- Solid tumors, lymphomas, leukemia

Cyclophosphamide

Cyclophosphamide

- Prodrug: Requires bioactivation by liver
  - Converted to phosphoramide mustard
  - Metabolized by liver P450 system

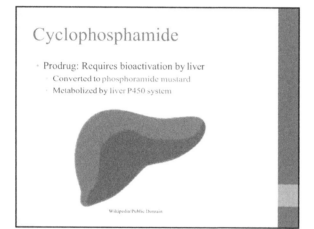

Wikipedia/Public Domain

Cyclophosphamide

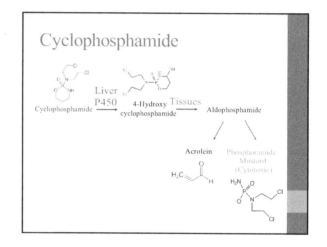

Cyclophosphamide → Liver P450 → 4-Hydroxy cyclophosphamide → Tissues → Aldophosphamide

Acrolein

Phosphoramide Mustard (Cytotoxic)

Cyclophosphamide
Side Effects

Mesna

- Myelosuppression
  - ↓WBC, ↓Hct, ↓Plt
- Hemorrhagic cystitis
  - Acrolein metabolite toxic to bladder
  - Hematuria +/- dysuria
  - Lower risk with hydration and mesna
  - Mesna: sodium 2-mercaptoethane sulfonate
  - Mesna binds and inactivates acrolein in the urine

Cyclophosphamide
Side Effects

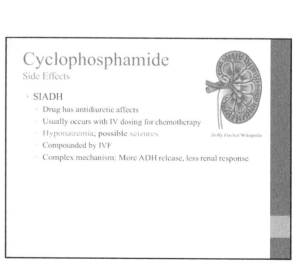

- SIADH
  - Drug has antidiuretic affects
  - Usually occurs with IV dosing for chemotherapy
  - Hyponatremia; possible seizures
  - Compounded by IVF
  - Complex mechanism: More ADH release, less renal response

Holly Fischer/Wikipedia

126

Ifosfamide

- Isomer of cyclophosphamide
- Used in germ cell cancer and sarcomas
- May also cause hemorrhagic cystitis

Ifosfamide

Ifosfamide

- Special side effect: nephrotoxicity
  - Toxic to proximal tubular cells
  - May cause Fanconi syndrome
  - Polyuria
  - Electrolyte losses: Hypokalemia, hypophosphatemia
  - Metabolic acidosis (loss of bicarb in urine)
- Special side effect: encephalopathy
  - 10-30% of patients

Ifosfamide

Nitrosoureas

Carmustine
bis-chloroethylnitrosourea
BCNU

Lomustine
chloroethylnitrosourea
CCNU

Streptozotocin

Semustine

Nitrosoureas

- Bioactivated in liver
- Highly lipid soluble ⬜ cross blood-brain barrier
- Used for brain tumors (glioblastoma multiforme)

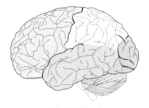

Wikipedia/Public Domain

Nitrosoureas
Toxicity

- Myelosuppression
- Rarely leads to pulmonary fibrosis
- Rarely chronic interstitial nephritis (renal failure)
- Encephalopathy and seizures
  - Very high dosages (BCNU for bone marrow transplant)

Busulfan

- Myeloablation
  - Single, high-dose of Busulfan
  - Results in severe pancytopenia (bone marrow ablation)
  - Preparation for stem cell transplant
- Chronic myeloid leukemia (CML)

Busulfan
Toxicity

- Myelosuppression
- Skin hyperpigmentation
  - Also occurs with other chemotherapy (Bleomycin)
- Seizures (high dosages)

Busulfan
Toxicity

- Pulmonary toxicity
  - Cough, dyspnea
  - Can progress to pulmonary fibrosis
  - Ground glass opacities
  - Restrictive PFTs
  - Reduced DLCO

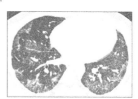

Dacarbazine

- Part of ABVD protocol for Hodgkin lymphoma
  - Adriamycin (doxorubicin) - cytotoxic antibiotics
  - Bleomycin - cytotoxic antibiotics
  - Vinblastine – microtubule inhibitor
  - Dacarbazine – alkylating agent

Procarbazine

- Part of MOPP protocol for Hodgkin lymphoma
  - Mechlorethamine – Mustard agent
  - Oncovin (Vincristine) – Microtubule drug
  - Procarbazine
  - Prednisone

Antitumor Antibiotics

Jason Ryan, MD, MPH

Antitumor Antibiotics

- Drugs derived from Streptomyces bacterial strains
- Anthracyclines

- Bleomycin

Anthracyclines

- Key drugs: daunorubicin and doxorubicin
- Others: idarubicin, epirubicin, mitoxantrone

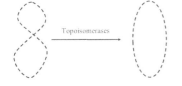

Daunorubicin   Doxorubicin
                      (Adriamycin)

Anthracyclines

- Multiple toxic mechanisms
  - Inhibition of topoisomerase II ☐ DNA breaks
  - Intercalation of DNA ☐ blocks synthesis of DNA/RNA
  - Generation of free radicals
- Cell cycle non-specific

Topoisomerase II

- Cuts both strands of DNA helix then reseals
- Relieves tangles and supercoils
- Anthracycline inhibition ☐ breaks with no resealing
- Result: DNA damage

Topoisomerases →

DNA Intercalation

- Binds to DNA
- Inserts between base pairs
- Inhibits replication/transcription

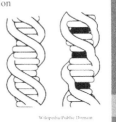

Wikipedia/Public Domain

Free Radicals

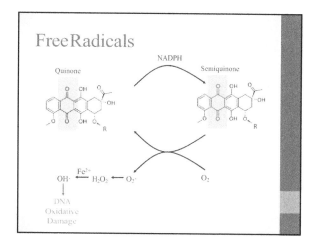

Anthracyclines
Clinical Uses

- Doxorubicin (Adriamycin)
  - Widely used anticancer drug
  - Breast cancer
  - Many solid tumors
  - Childhood cancers: neuroblastoma, Ewing's, osteosarcoma
  - Leukemia/lymphoma

Anthracyclines
Cardiotoxicity

- Systolic heart failure (↓LVEF)
- Free radical damage to myocytes ☐ necrosis
- Can present with dyspnea, fatigue, edema
- Screening: echocardiogram after infusions

Anthracyclines
Cardiotoxicity

- Rarely seen with lower total dosages
- Dexrazoxane
  - Iron chelating agent
  - Limits anthracycline-induced cardiotoxicity

Dactinomycin
Actinomycin D

- Several mechanisms
  - Intercalates in DNA
  - Inhibits RNA synthesis (transcription)
  - Double strand breaks
- Childhood cancers
  - Neuroblastoma, Ewing's sarcoma, osteosarcoma
- Major adverse effect: myelosuppression

Bleomycin

- Binds to DNA
- Free radical formation (oxygen, iron)
- Single and double strand breaks
- Cell cycle-specific drug: accumulates in G2 phase

Zephyris /Wikipedia

Bleomycin
Clinical Uses

- Lymphomas
- Germ cell tumors
- Head and neck cancer
- Squamous cell cancer of skin
- Cancers of cervix and vulva

Bleomycin
Toxicity

- Inactivated by enzyme bleomycin hydrolase
- Lower enzyme activity in skin and lungs
- Skin toxicity
  - Many skin changes described
  - Also seen with other chemotherapy drugs (Busulfan)
  - "Flagellate erythema": Red/dark streaks on skin

Bleomycin
Pulmonary Toxicity

- Dose-limiting adverse effect
- Usually presents as pneumonitis
  - Cough, dyspnea, crackles
  - Infiltrates on chest X-ray
- Risk factors
  - Older patients (>70)
  - Prior pulmonary disease

Microtubule Inhibitors

Jason Ryan, MD, MPH

Microtubules

- Polymers of α and β tubulin
- Can grow/collapse
- Flagella, cilia, cellular transport (axons)

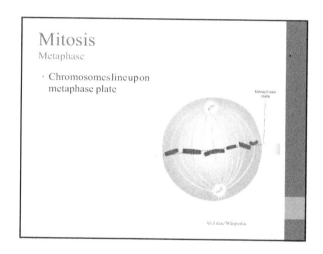

Thomas Splettstoesser (www.scistyle.com)

Mitosis

- Part of cell cycle
- Separation of chromosomes for cell division
- Depends heavily on microtubules (mitotic spindle)
- Followed by cytokinesis: cell divides

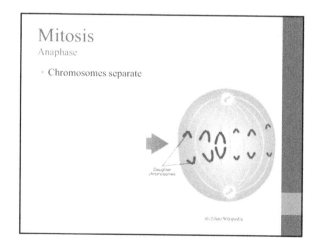

Lordjuppiter /Wikipedia

Mitosis
Metaphase

- Chromosomes line up on metaphase plate

Ali Zifan/Wikipedia

Mitosis
Anaphase

- Chromosomes separate

Ali Zifan/Wikipedia

Cell Cycle

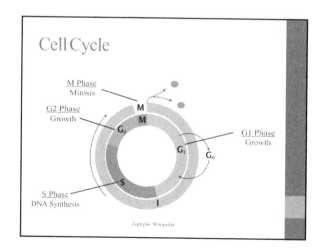

Zephyris -Wikipedia

Microtubule Inhibitors

- Taxols
- Vinca alkaloids

Vocabulary

- Alkaloids
  - Naturally occurring substances
  - Nitrogen-containing bases
  - Usually derived from plants or trees

Nicotine
(Tobacco)

Morphine
(Opium)

Taxols
Paclitaxel, Docetaxel

- Alkaloids from yew trees
- Mitotic spindle poisons
- Bind microtubules
- Enhance tubulin polymerization
- Microtubules cannot break down
- Blocks cell cycle at metaphase/anaphase transition
- Anaphase cannot occur

Taxols
Clinical Use

- Solid tumors
  - Ovarian and breast cancer
  - Non-small cell and small cell lung cancer
  - Head and neck cancers
  - Prostate and bladder cancer

Taxols
Toxicity

- Hypersensitivity reactions (up to 30% patients)
  - Dyspnea/wheezing
  - Urticaria
  - Hypotension
- Premedication often used for prevention
  - Glucocorticoids and antihistamines
- Nabpaclitaxel (Abraxane)
  - Albumin-bound paclitaxel
  - Lower risk hypersensitivity reactions
  - Premedication not required

James Heilman, MD

Taxols
Toxicity

- Myelosuppression
- Neuropathy
  - Sensory nerves
  - Usually burning paresthesias of hands/feet

Vinca Alkaloids
Vincristine, vinblastine

- Derived from periwinkle plant (Vinca rosea)
- Bind β-tubulin
- Inhibit polymerization
- Prevent spindle formation
- Mitotic arrest in metaphase

Vinca Alkaloids
Clinical Uses

- Breast cancer
- Germ cell cancer
- Lymphomas
- ABVD Protocol (Hodgkin lymphoma)
  - Adriamycin (doxorubicin) - cytotoxic antibiotics
  - Bleomycin - cytotoxic antibiotics
  - Vinblastine
  - Dacarbazine – alkylating agent

Vinca Alkaloids
Toxicity

- Myelosuppression
- SIADH (rare)
- Vincristine: Neurotoxicity
  - Dose-limiting toxicity
  - Loss of axonal transport
  - Sensory and motor
  - Paresthesias/pain in fingers and feet
  - Distal weakness

DNA Drugs

Jason Ryan, MD, MPH

DNA Drugs

- Antitumor Antibiotics
- Alkylating agents
- Platinum agents
- Topoisomerase I and II inhibitors

Platinum Agents
Cisplatin, carboplatin, oxaliplatin

- Cross link DNA similar to alkylating agents
  - Most commonly at N7 nitrogen of guanine
  - "Alkylating like" drugs
  - Cell cycle nonspecific (like alkylating agents)

Cisplatin

Platinum Agents
Clinical Uses

- Solid tumors
  - Non-small cell and small cell lung cancer
  - Esophageal and gastric cancer
  - Head and neck cancers
  - Testicular cancer
  - Ovarian cancer

Platinum Agents
Toxicity

- All can cause neuropathy
  - Usually a peripheral sensory neuropathy
  - Pain, burning, tingling
  - Often in feet or hands
- May also cause ototoxicity (hearing loss)
- GI distress (nausea/vomiting) up to 90% patients

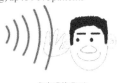

Pixabay/Public Domain

Platinum Agents
Nephrotoxicity

- Main, dose-limiting side effect of cisplatin
  - Often presents as acute kidney injury (↑BUN/Cr)
  - Prevented with IV fluids (normal saline)
  - Increase urine output (cause diuresis)
  - Amifostine: Free radical scavenger
  - Used in ovarian cancer with repeated cisplatin doses
- Carboplatin: less renal toxicity

Amifostine

Topoisomerases

- Relieve tangles and supercoils in DNA
- Cuts strands of DNA helix then reseal
- Chemotherapy inhibition □ breaks with no resealing
- Result: DNA damage
- Affect S/G2 phase (during/after DNA synthesis)

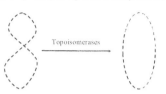

Topoisomerases

Topoisomerases

- Topoisomerase I
  - Breaks single strands of DNA then reseals
- Topoisomerase II
  - Breaks double strands of DNA then reseals

Topoisomerase I Inhibitors
Irinotecan, topotecan

- "Camptothecins"
- From Camptotheca ("happy tree") tree in China

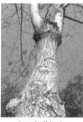

Geographer/Wikipedia

Topoisomerase I Inhibitors
Clinical Uses

- Irinotecan
  - Colon Cancer
- Topotecan
  - Ovarian cancer
  - Small cell lung cancer

Topoisomerase I Inhibitors
Toxicity

- Myelosuppression
- Severe diarrhea
  - Risk of volume depletion

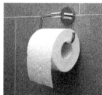

Elya/Wikipedia

Topoisomerase II Inhibitors
Etoposide, teniposide

- Synthesized from Podophyllotoxins
- Derived from May apple plant (Podophyllum)

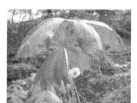

Wikipedia Public Domain

Topoisomerase II Inhibitors
Clinical Use

- Intravenous and oral
- Germ cell cancers
- Small cell and non-small cell lung cancer
- Lymphomas
- Main toxicity: Myelosuppression, nausea/vomiting

Other Cancer Drugs

Jason Ryan, MD, MPH

Monoclonal Antibodies

- Laboratory-produced antibody
- Derived from cloned cells in culture

- Administered by intravenous infusion

Martin Brändli /Wikipedia

Infusion Reactions

- Usually occur after 1st or 2nd infusion
- Antibody-antigen binding ☐ cytokine release
- Most are mild to moderate
- Fever/chills
- Flushing and itching
- Skin rashes
- Nausea, vomiting, and/or diarrhea
- Treatment/prevention: antihistamines, steroids

Bevacizumab
Avastin

- Monoclonal antibody to VEGF-A
- Prevents VEGF-A from binding VEGF receptors
- Used in many solid tumors
  - Colorectal cancer
  - Breast
  - Renal cell carcinoma

Martin Brändli /Wikipedia

VEGF
Vascular endothelial growth factor

- Family of signal proteins
- Several forms (VEGF-A/B/C/D)
- VEGF-A: Stimulates angiogenesis
- Secreted by tumors ☐ vascular growth
- VEGF Inhibitors
  - Bevacizumab (cancer)
  - Ranibizumab (retinopathy)

Bevacizumab
Toxicity

- VEGF mediates vasodilation via nitric oxide
- Inhibition ☐ vasoconstriction
- Cardiovascular adverse effects
  - Hypertension
  - Increased risk of arterial thromboembolism
  - Myocardial infarction/stroke/TIA
- Other effects
  - Delayed wound healing
  - Bleeding

EGF

Epidermal growth factor

- Stimulates cell growth and differentiation
- Binds to EGFR
  - Tyrosine kinase receptor
  - EGF-EGFR binding □ phosphorylation of tyrosine residues
  - Phosphorylated EGFR □ downstream effects
- EGFR overexpressed in many tumors

Tyrosine

EGFR

Wikipedia/Public Domain

Cetuximab

- Monoclonal antibody
- Binds extracellular domain of EGFR
- Blocks binding of EGF-EGFR
- Solid tumors
  - Non-small cell lung cancer
  - Colon cancer
  - Head and neck cancer
- Side effects in clinical trial:
  - Rash (acne)
  - Diarrhea

Martin Brändli -Wikipedia

KRAS Mutation

Colorectal Cancer

- K-ras
  - G-protein
  - Downstream of EGFR
  - Can acquire activating mutations in colon cancer
  - Mutations isolate tumor cells from effect of EGFR
- Mutated K-ras: No benefit from cetuximab
- Wild-type K-ras: Cetuximab beneficial

K-ras mutations and benefit from cetuximab in advanced colorectal cancer. N Engl J Med. 2008 Oct 23;359(17):1757-65.

Erlotinib

Tarceva

- EGFR tyrosine kinase inhibitor (oral)
- Major use: non-small cell lung cancer

Erlotinib

Tarceva

- Main adverse effect: Skin rash
  - Acne-like eruption
  - Upper torso, face, neck
  - May be an indicator of drug effect
  - Seen with all EGFR-blocking drugs (Cetuximab)

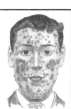

Wikipedia/Public Domain

Imatinib
Tyrosine Kinase Inhibitor

- Chronic myeloid leukemia
  - Philadelphia chromosome/BCR-ABL fusion gene
  - Tyrosine kinase protein
  - Treatment: Imatinib
  - Also other TKIs: dasatinib, nilotinib, bosutinib

Imatinib
Tyrosine Kinase Inhibitor

- Gastrointestinal stromal tumors (GIST)
  - Rare stomach and small intestine tumors
  - Associated with c-KIT mutations
  - Treatment: surgery +/- Imatinib

KIT Mutations

- KIT (c-KIT) protein
  - Found on cell surface (CD117)
  - Tyrosine kinase receptor
  - Binds KIT ligand (stem cell factor)
  - Stimulates growth
- KIT mutations □ cancer (proto-oncogene)
- KIT gain-of-function mutations in 95% GIST
  - CD117 positive cells

Imatinib
Adverse Effects

- Fluid retention
  - Usually peripheral or periobital edema
  - Sometimes pulmonary edema
- Rash

Klaus D. Peter,   James Heilman, MD/Wikipedia

Rituximab

- Monoclonal CD20 antibody
- Leads to depletion of B cells
- Used in B-cell malignancy and autoimmune diseases

Martin Brändli /Wikipedia

Rituximab

- B-cell malignancies
  - Non-Hodgkin lymphoma
  - Chronic lymphocytic leukemia
- Rheumatoid arthritis
- Immune thrombocytopenia (ITP)
  - First line therapy: IVIG and steroids
  - 2nd line therapy: splenectomy
  - Alternative: Rituximab

Rituximab
Toxicity

- Rare cases of opportunistic infections
  - Pneumocystis jirovecii pneumonia
  - Cryptococcal meningitis
  - Cytomegalovirus colitis
  - Progressive multifocal leukoencephalopathy (JC virus)
- Hepatitis B reactivation

Tamoxifen

- Selective estrogen receptor modulator (SERM)
- Oral drug
- Competitive antagonist of breast estrogen receptor
  - Used in ER positive (ER+) breast cancer
  - Used as part of primary therapy
  - Also used for prevention

Tamoxifen

- Estrogen agonist in other tissues (bone/uterus)
- Bone: Estrogen increases bone density
- Uterus: Estrogen promotes endothelial growth

Tamoxifen
Toxicity

- Hot flashes (estrogen blockade)
- Increased risk of DVT/PE
  - Estrogen effects ⁻increased clotting factors

DVT/PE

Tamoxifen
Toxicity

- Partial agonist to endometrium
  - Endometrial proliferation
  - Hyperplasia
  - Polyp formation
- May cause endometrial cancer
  - Associated with invasive carcinoma and uterine sarcoma
- Major risk in postmenopausal women

Raloxifene
Evista

- Also a SERM
- Estrogen actions on bone
- Anti-estrogen in breast/uterus
- Osteoporosis (postmenopausal women)
- Also used for prevention of breast cancer
- May cause hot flashes
- Associated with DVT/PE

Aromatase Inhibitors
Anastrozole, Letrozole, Exemestane

- ER+ breast cancer – postmenopausal women
- Block estrogen production
  - Peripheral tissues
  - Also occurs in breast cancer cells
- Inhibit aromatase enzyme
  - Androstenedione ⊓ estrone
  - Testosterone ⊓ estradiol

Anastrozole

Letrozole

Exemestane (steroid)

Aromatase Inhibitors
Adverse Effects

- Osteoporosis (loss of estrogen)
- Increased risk of fracture

Open Stax College

Trastuzumab
Herceptin

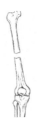

- Monoclonal antibody to HER-2
  - Surface receptor
  - Activation ⊓ cell growth and proliferation
  - Overexpressed by cancer cells
  - Expressed in 25 to 30% of breast cancers
- Many names for HER2
  - HER2/neu
  - ERB2
  - CD340

Martin Brändli /Wikipedia

HER Family

- Human epithelial receptors
- All have inner tyrosine kinase domain
- Activation ⊓ signaling cascade ⊓ growth

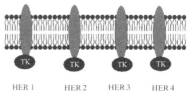

HER 1   HER 2   HER 3   HER 4
EGFR

Trastuzumab
Herceptin

- Improves survival in breast cancer
  - Inhibits proliferation of tumor cells
  - Antibody-dependent cell-mediated cytotoxicity

Satchmo2000/Wikipedia

Trastuzumab
Toxicity

- Cardiomyopathy
  - Usually asymptomatic ↓ LVEF
  - May lead to heart failure (dyspnea, fatigue, edema)
- Most likely due to blockade of HER2 in myocytes
  - May lead to stunning of myocardium
- Different from anthracycline cardiotoxicity
  - Not dose dependent
  - Often reversible when drug discontinued
  - Re-challenge often tolerated after LVEF recovery
  - Biopsy: No necrosis

Porphyrias

Jason Ryan, MD, MPH

Porphyrins

- Large nitrogen-containing molecules
- Porphyrias = disorders of porphyrin synthesis
- All from deficient enzymes in heme synthesis
- Rarely cause anemia
- Symptoms from accumulation of porphyrins

Protoporphyrin   Heme

Heme

- Component of hemoglobin
- Mostly produced in bone marrow and liver
- Bone marrow: 80% of heme production
  - Used in red blood cells as hemoglobin
- Liver: 20% heme production
  - Used in cytochrome P450 enzymes

Heme

Heme Synthesis

- Begins in mitochondria
  - Initial ingredients: Succinyl CoA and glycine
  - Combined to form δ-ALA (delta-aminolevulinic acid)
  - Enzyme: δ-ALA synthase
  - Rate limiting step (inhibited by heme)
- Middle pathway in cytosol
- Final steps in mitochondria

Heme Synthesis

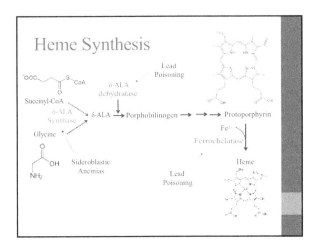

Heme Synthesis

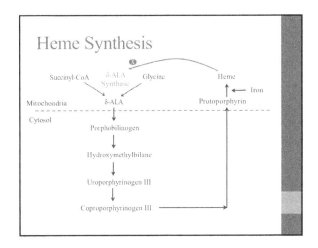

Porphyrias

- More than eight different types described
- Two most common (all rare):
  - Porphyria cutanea tarda
  - Acute intermittent porphyria
- Both do not cause anemia (no ↓ hemoglobin)
- Symptoms from accumulation of intermediates

Porphyria Cutanea Tarda

- Most common porphyria
- Deficient activity of UROD
  - Uroporphyrinogen decarboxylase
  - 5th enzyme in heme synthesis pathway

Porphyria Cutanea Tarda

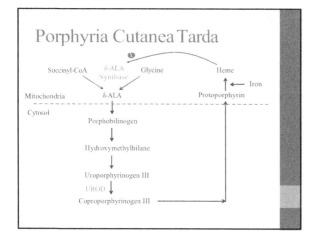

Vocabulary

- Uroporphyrinogens:
  - Four propionic acid groups (3 carbons)
  - Four acetic acid groups (2 carbons)
- Different arrangements in I versus III
- Uroporphyrinogen III more common form
- Forms II, IV do not occur naturally

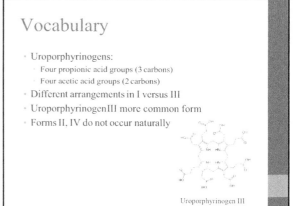

Uroporphyrinogen III

Vocabulary

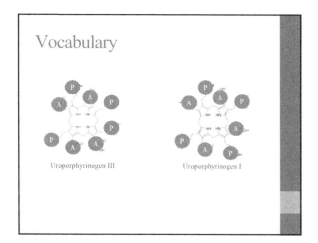

Uroporphyrinogen III   Uroporphyrinogen I

Vocabulary

- "Porphyrinogen" = non-oxidized molecule
- "Porphyrin" = oxidized molecule (loss of hydrogen)

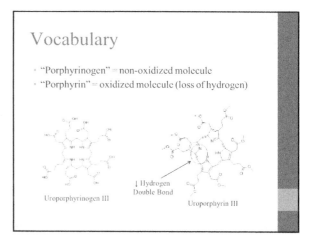

Uroporphyrinogen III

↓ Hydrogen
Double Bond

Uroporphyrin III